DATE DUE

Understanding Health Care Reform

Understanding Health Care Reform

THEODORE R. MARMOR

YALE UNIVERSITY PRESS
NEW HAVEN AND LONDON

Set in Times Roman type by DEKR Corp., Woburn, Massachusetts.
Printed in the United States of America by Vail-Ballou Press, Binghamton, New York.

Library of Congress Cataloging-in-Publication Data

Marmor, Theodore R.
    Understanding health care reform / Theodore R. Marmor.
       p. cm.
    Includes bibliographical references and index.
    ISBN 0-300-05878-0 (acid-free paper). — ISBN 0-300-05879-9 (pbk.
: acid-free paper)
      1. Health care reform—United States. 2. Medical care—United
States—Cost control. 3. Insurance, Health—United States.
I. Title.
RA395.A3M378 1994   94-15886
362.1′0973—dc   CIP

A catalogue record of this book is available from the British Library.

The paper in this book meets the guidelines for permanence and durability of the Committee on Production Guidelines for Book Longevity of the Council on Library Resources.

10 9 8 7 6 5 4 3 2 1

For Jerry Mashaw

Contents

Preface

The essays that make up this book reflect my reform aspirations, but they do not constitute a reformer's brief. Rather, they represent years of effort to understand the dynamics of American medicine, the political constraints that shape our policies, and the lessons that history and comparative study can offer. They reflect as well the conviction that nations do not solve socioeconomic problems with panaceas. At best, collectivities learn to cope better with the more or less intractable conflicts among objectives, interests, and limited resources and opportunities.

Proceeding from that premise, these collected writings address the institutional constraints on our capacity to reform American medicine: the legacy of our history, the character of the ordinary politics that shape fields of medical policymaking, the unusual opportunity provided by a consensus on the severity of our troubles, and the familiar risks that a fragmented polity will confuse the doable with the desirable.

Following an introductory chapter, Part I of this book addresses both how the health reform debate emerged in American politics and what shapes the politics of particularly contentious health policy issues.

Chapter 2 explicitly takes up the question of how we got to where we are. It characterizes the long road to reform, emphasizing the extent to which we are debating today the same issues that emerged in the so-called health crisis of the early 1970s. Published in part to contest complacent views of American medicine, it highlights the long history of American medical inflation and the worldwide attention to rising health expenditures ever since the fiscal strains of stagflation emerged in the wake of the oil crisis of 1973–1974. It locates the American political debate in the context of an international struggle to contain medical costs amid economic troubles and a heightened and widespread skepticism about government's capacity to right social wrongs.

The chapter also emphasizes some of the peculiarities of American politics in its handling of common strains. These include the fragmented nature of our political system, the persistent pattern of searching for policy panaceas that always disappoint, and the development since the mid-1970s of so-called competitive models of a rationalized system of medical care finance and delivery. It sets the stage for explaining how the Clinton election galvanized reform forces that had been building for years.

The remaining four essays in this part take up the varied politics of particular medical care issues. Chapter 3 summarizes the common and distinctive ways in which international economic strains affected major public programs, including medical care. Chapter 4 discusses the important role the nonprofits have played in American medicine and the evidence that bears on the contentions of critics and admirers. Chapter 5 takes up a particularly revealing example of the American disposition to oscillate between idealistic searches for a medical panacea and subsequent disappointment. It critically appraises the argument that much of American medical care is wasteful and that cutting out that waste—through utilization review, more scientific evidence on "outcomes," and the like—is some sort of magic bullet of cost control. Chapter 6 reviews an influential book by Henry Aaron and William Schwartz on the lessons of British rationing for the reform of American medicine. It skeptically examines the relevance of the very different context of British medical politics and discusses the difficulties Americans have both in addressing rationing decisions soberly and in learning from the extensive experience of others with regard to acceptable forms of allocating medical care and controlling costs.

Part II turns more directly to the debate over universal health insurance. Chapter 7 concentrates on the subordination of realistic forecasts of implementation to ideologically charged claims about the merits of one or another version of health insurance reform. It emphasizes the gap between naive panaceas and cynical assumptions of intractability, noting how useful it would be to make our choices depend on what plans would be like in practice rather than on what they are labeled in theory.

Chapter 8 elaborates on the theme of implementation in connection with arguments for and against using more price-competitive insurance markets to reform this country's medical troubles. It underlines how little practical experience is available for resting reform on such models. But the chapter also discusses the extraordinarily substantial impact of the language and values of competitive markets on the national debate over health reform. This discussion is of obvious relevance to the efforts of contemporary reformers—President Clinton included—to find some compromise between the instruments of markets and those of governments in reforming our medical care practices.

Chapter 9 presents my own remedial ideas and assesses the fears that have bedeviled attempts of a reasoned debate over what course of reform action to take. Originally a speech to an annual meeting of medical specialists, the essay is more restrained here than in the form published by *Lear's* magazine in the winter of 1993.

Chapter 10 asks why since the Clinton election there has been such a truncated discussion of the Canadian model of universal health insurance. Though overwhelmingly popular in Canada and in the early 1970s one of the leading models of reform in the United States, so-called single-payer reform plans were practically pushed off the table of discussion by a curious combination of journalistic, congressional, and presidential presumptions. The chapter tries to explain how and why that happened. It clearly reflects the disappointment of the coauthors in that development, but concentrates on explanation, not advocacy. Chapter 11 takes as its subject the persistent tendency in American politics to move back and forth between simpleminded panaceas and dreary pessimism. The health reform debate well illustrates one way in which American managerial thought has obscured the real choices in reform: namely, the suggestion that the newest in managerial fads— managed competition—will magically right the wrongs of American medicine. Chapter 11 places this view and others like it in the context of changing fashions of corporate thought over the past quarter-century: the world of centralization and then decentralization, conglomerates and then the opposite, hard-edged competitiveness and then quality circles, and so on.

Part III, on comparative perspectives, presents two essays on what can and cannot be properly learned from international experience with universal health insurance. Chapter 12 is an extensive discussion of the Canadian experience with national health insurance. It not only discusses the political uses to which claims about Canada have been put, but also summarizes what has really been going on in Canada since the early 1970s. Chapter 13 is quite different, a short essay on the nature of the Japanese population's remarkable improvement in health status since World War II, the challenges to the quality of its medical care, and the relevance of that paradox for American debates about insurance reform and health promotion. An expert on Canada and an amateur on Japan, I have included this piece for whatever stimulation it can offer as we think of foreign experience rather than for its scholarly authoritativeness.

Part IV concentrates on the more immediate politics of health insurance reform in the post-1992 period. The discussion in Chapter 14 comments on an issue that has been largely buried under the torrent of words about the Clinton reform effort: namely, how will the Medicare program be treated in any version of universal health insurance? The chapter makes a case for taking this matter seriously, especially in light of the unexpected controversy about catastrophic coverage under Medicare in the 1987–1989 period.

The concluding chapter brings together concerns about the workability of various reform proposals. It proceeds from earlier discussions and concentrates on how implementation should affect one's evaluation of reform options. The most recent of my published works on health reform, its theme will be relevant to whatever policy choices emerge in the course of this decade.

These essays, as is clear from the coauthors cited, are as much collective as individual efforts. They are almost wholly contemporary pieces, but they reflect a long history of collaboration with a number of writers. Some coauthors—Jan Blustein, David Boyum, and Carlos Cano—are former students of mine who are now scholars in their own right. Others—Mark Goldberg, Tom Hamburger, Rudolf Klein, and Jerry Mashaw—are widely recognized colleagues whose work I have drawn on with might appear promiscuous ease. They (and I) recognize the personal and scholarly interdependence, and it would be churlish to slight the degree to which this is collaborative work. This is most prominently the case with Jerry Mashaw, my closest Yale colleague and the one with whom I have written most frequently. Having coauthored one book on *America's Misunderstood Welfare State,* coedited another on *Social Security,* and together written numerous articles, we are undeniably a scholarly team. In that respect, this book's merits are very much joint and I want to acknowledge the enormous debt I owe this capable friend, while freeing him of responsibility for what he did not write.

Others have contributed in ways that can easily be overlooked. Elizabeth Auld, for the 1980s my aide and now a practicing physician's assistant, helped to bring many of these essays to fruition. Bob Gribbons and John Pakutka, my former students at Yale's School of Organization and Management, were very valuable research assistants between 1991 and 1993. And so was Michael Barr, then a student at the Yale Law School and my coauthor on a longer paper that is the basis of much of the first chapter. Jon Oberlander, a doctoral student in political science at Yale, has turned into an exceedingly reliable research assistant and assisted with more of these essays than is formally noted. My assistant, Lynn Murinson, helped with the usual tasks, but did so with unusual good humor and competence.

The Henry J. Kaiser Family Foundation, in a generous grant for health policy studies at Yale's School of Organization and Management, made financially possible not only scholarly research but a faculty-student workshop that has greatly enriched the intellectual environment in which I and others have worked. In 1987 the Canadian Institute for Advanced Research awarded me a five-year fellowship that largely freed me from ordinary teaching and administrative responsibilities. This grant provided not only the freedom to pursue my writing but colleagues in the institute's program in population health who greatly stimulated by work. My gratitude to the institute's president, J. Fraser Mustard, and to colleagues in the health program—particularly its director, Bob Evans—is literally immense. And Yale's Institution for Social and Policy Studies, headed now by Bradford Gray, has been a welcome interdisciplinary part of my professional environment. Finally, a word of thanks to another Yale colleague, Robert Burt, a friend who critically commented on more of these essays than his schedule or judgment should have permitted. My gratitude to all of these persons and institutions is substantial, though with the usual disclaimers of responsibility for the scholarly products they facilitated but did not write.

Chapter 1
American Health Care Reform: Separating Sense from Nonsense

WITH MARK GOLDBERG

The reform of American medical care has been, since at least the fall of 1991, at the very top of the nation's political agenda. Precisely how and why that came to be is not self-evident. After all, Americans had been told for more than two decades that our medical system was in crisis. Polling studies show that most citizens accepted this view long before the nation's political leaders began offering up serious plans for fundamental reform.[1] Moreover, while medical inflation outdistanced general consumer price increases in the early 1990s, the gap was even wider during the first Reagan administration, when, according to the conventional political wisdom, universal health insurance was unthinkable.[2]

One of us (T.R.M.) speaks from experience on this matter, having been the senior social policy adviser to Walter Mondale during the 1984 presidential campaign. Literally no one in that campaign thought it possible to discuss national health insurance, although the rising cost of medical care was a theme in the Mondale campaign's attack on President Reagan.

The question of why major reform is not only thinkable now but the major domestic preoccupation of the Clinton administration has many answers, none of them simple. The end of the cold war and the exaltation over the 1991 military triumph in Iraq made domestic issues by

1

Table 1.1
Comparison of the change in total health care expenditures in several
countries

Country	1970 (% of GDP[a])	1980 (% of GDP)	1990 (% of GDP)	Percent increase, 1980–1990
United States	7.4	9.3	12.4	33.3
Canada	7.1	7.4	9.0	21.6
Germany	5.9	8.5	8.1	−4.7
France	5.8	7.6	8.9	17.1
Sweden	7.2	9.5	8.7	−8.4
Italy	5.2	6.8	7.6	11.8
Japan	4.4	6.4	6.5	1.5
Britain	4.5	5.8	6.1	4.7

a. GDP = Gross Domestic Product.
Sources: U.S. Health Care Financing Administration; Organization for
Economic Cooperation and Development.

the late spring of 1991 far more salient. Hospitals awash in red ink,
workers locked into jobs for fear of losing access to health insurance,
fraudulent billing practices by some hospitals, doctors, and laboratories,
nightmarish stories of uninsured persons driven into bankruptcy—all
were part of the medical care commentary of the early 1990s. Moreover,
as Table 1.1 and Figure 1.1 demonstrate, the cost of health care has
risen relentlessly, and most dramatically, in the United States, where
in 1991 we spent $2,868 for each citizen on health care. At the same
time, Americans without health insurance now number about 37 million,
which in 1992 included over 10 million children, 6 million unemployed,
and 5 million part-time workers. A person who works in construction,
personal services, or agriculture, as Figure 1.2 shows, has a far greater
likelihood of not having health insurance; on average, a shocking 17
percent of all working people in the United States have no health
insurance.

But it was the presidential race of 1992—and the presence of a
Democratic challenger committed to reforming American medicine—
that made the medical care problems of the country front-page news.
In that context, a 1992 bidding war over policy remedies was inevitable:

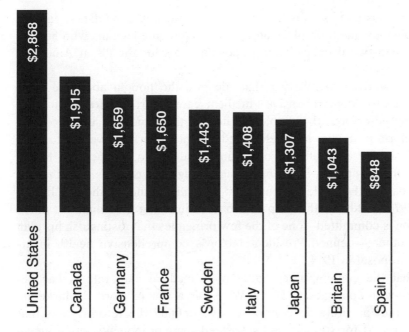

Figure 1.1 A comparison of health spending: the amount spent in various countries for each citizen on health care, 1991, in U.S. dollars. (Source: Organization for Economic Cooperation and Development.)

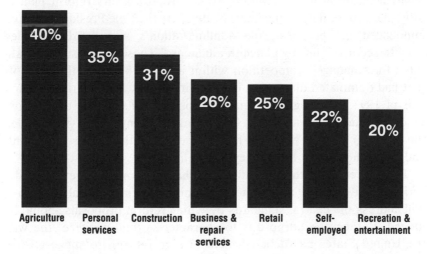

Figure 1.2 Job sectors in the United States with higher-than-average percentages of uninsured employees, 1991.

one obvious contest was between the presidential candidates; another less obvious one took place among the policy intellectuals who had for more than two decades been proposing cures for the ills of American medicine.

It is worth remembering that, despite the hoopla about new approaches to "comprehensive" medical care reform, there is virtually nothing new about the problems cited or the remedies suggested. All the reform principles now celebrated—from universal coverage to fixed physician fee schedules, from global budgets to competitive health plans, from employer-based financing to single-payer plans,[3] and more— were part of the battle over national health insurance in the first half of the 1970s. Indeed, the employer-based financing to which President Clinton is committed—one of the few principles that distinguish his plan from others—defined President Nixon's comprehensive health insurance proposal in 1974.[4]

What the contemporary battle over medical care reform has become—with apologies to H. G. Wells—is a war of words.[5] Marketing labels (not accurate descriptions) have defined the reform plans that have jousted for support and separated their proponents into warring camps in the period since Harris Wofford's startling Senate victory over Richard Thornburgh in Pennsylvania in November of 1991. The most prominent camps came to be labeled by the reform slogans of single-payer, play-or-pay, and managed competition.

At least that was the case until media attention came to focus on what the Clinton administration would propose as its reform plan in May (then June, then September) of 1993. By the time President Clinton announced his proposal, the administration's war words included "health security" through "health alliances." These expressions substituted for "managed competition within a global budget," the symbols that had dominated discussion in the Clinton task force during the first half of 1993. Focus groups, and Clinton polling experts, finally convinced the administration that the "managed competition" label failed the marketer's test. The public hardly knew what the expression meant; and when they heard more, they didn't like it.

The objective of this introductory chapter is not, however, to describe or to evaluate the Clinton administration's proposal, though it will address the central standards by which reform proposals should be judged. Rather, the purpose is to characterize (and criticize) the way the United States has debated medical care reform, to suggest some ground rules for doing better, and to bring to bear on that debate information about the implementation of any major reform that proponents should be forced to consider. American politics, we know from the struggles over federal aid to education, civil rights, Medicare, and AIDS, addresses major reform questions in fits and starts.

The fragmentation of American politics makes the process of reform uncertain. But the contemporary combination of presidential commitment, congressional readiness to act, and what might be called the public's permissive consensus about bold reform does not often arise. So it is worth attending to the gap between the likelihood of reform and the real possibility that reform will not work well over time. Unless the debate reflects an understanding of our historical legacy and the dangers of provincial naivete, we risk mythical mismatches between problem and remedy. And unless the debate—and the congressional decisions— address implementation questions adequately, we also risk squandering a remarkable opportunity to right the wrongs of a system no one defends. Put another way, a consensus on wrongs does not assure anyone that programmatic reforms will right them.

We will proceed here as follows. The first section of this chapter briefly presents what we see as the lessons of previous attempts in twentieth-century American politics to enact universal health insurance. The second section discusses confusions within our contemporary debate, particularly the obfuscation that marketing labels entail as proponents and opponents jockey for advantage. The third section proposes some straightforward principles of evaluation that we believe should be applied to any proposal for universal health insurance. It suggests some ground rules for debate over the President's proposal and the alternatives offered. An avalanche of words followed in the wake of the Clinton task force's submission to the Congress in October 1993. How subsequent debate can be understood and elevated is our concern, though we are not so naive to think that the writing of health policy intellectuals will itself right the imbalance of our political debating practices. The last section takes up the question of what we know about narrowing the gap between what Americans want from reform and what the reformers propose. Here we draw on bodies of evidence and experience that no prudent actor responsible for results should ignore (or be permitted to ignore).

What President Clinton proposed could not possibly be specified in detail from his campaign promises. As a campaigner, he understandably avoided the details of health reform and its implementation. As President, he has different obligations, opportunities, and risks. The product of his unprecedented health task force in 1993 was but the beginning of a furious debate, one that thus far has concentrated more on labels for competing proposals than on substantive policy and political choices. Whether the President's plan—or an adjusted version of it—can command a majority of the Congress is even more problematic than the 1993 struggles over Clinton's deficit reduction plan and the North American Free Trade Agreement.

HISTORY: LESSON OR LAMENTATION?

The task of altering the way American medicine is financed is one of the most difficult a presidential reformer faces. At four other moments in twentieth-century American politics, reformers and their presidential backers tried. In the Progressive era, during the New Deal, under President Truman, and during the early 1970s, advocates thought universal health insurance was imminent and were bitterly disappointed. Now, as then, entrenched interests have tried to block national health insurance by skillfully manipulating our deepest fears to protect what they regard as their interests. In 1993, to be sure, these interest groups seemed on the defensive; the time for reform appeared to have arrived. But before the Clinton administration and the Congress can resolve the challenges of workable reform, they will have to resolve some of the nastiest ideological and budgetary conflicts in American politics. What can be learned by reviewing earlier efforts by presidents committed to reform but faced with seemingly intractable problems of substance, symbol, and support?

The health reformers of the Progressive era were convinced that broadened health insurance, financed and administered through social insurance, held the key to improved health, health care, and economic security. But theirs was an elite consensus, helped in the pre–World War I period by the apparent acquiescence of the American Medical Association (AMA). As it turned out, there was nothing like massive popular agreement on the need for change, and when the AMA turned against the idea, the reform movement withered. A negative consensus on the need for change, it appears, is a necessary but not a sufficient condition for successful reform.

The Lost Reform: Compulsory Health Insurance in the New Deal

The agony of the Great Depression generated enormous opportunities for change in American domestic policy. President Roosevelt led the way, commissioning expert group after expert group to take on the reforms needed in welfare, unemployment, agricultural failure, banking collapse, and in the institutions of economic security more generally.

The opening for universal health insurance came in 1935 with the famous Committee of Economic Security. A cabinet-level special committee, the CES took a year to review the circumstances of welfare, unemployment, child health, and old-age poverty, and to arrive at a package of programmatic suggestions. It did its work with admirable skill and timeliness, fashioning workable ideas from a far-flung research investigation of various methods of resolving these difficult problems. Unemployment and welfare were the most pressing issues; retirement benefits, though they have loomed much larger in subsequent decades, did not dominate the deliberations. In the matter of compulsory health insurance the President hesitated, worried that the presumed opposition of the American Medical Association and its ideological allies might jeopardize the success of the rest of his reform package. So it was that the committee refrained from even studying health insurance reform, leaving that to the congressional advocates who, in the next decade, would under the banner of the Murray-Wagner-Dingell bill frustratingly try to generate majority support.

From National Health Insurance to Medicare: The Dogged Retreat

President Truman's experience was no less frustrating. He fought the election battle of 1948 with national health insurance prominent among his proposals for a Fair Deal. But he faced, during the election and after, a barrage of ideological criticism that linked national health insurance with socialism, communism, and the recently demonized Soviet Union. After years of facing certain defeat in the Congress, Truman turned his executive advisers to a more modest goal: a health insurance program for social security recipients that would in time become the Medicare program of 1965. During Truman's presidency the general public was, according to the polls, always supportive of government health insurance. But this support was neither deep nor informed; socialized medicine was a tag that scared many, enough that no amount of presidential enthusiasm seemed adequate to assure support in the Congress. What we later came to know as the conservative coalition—linked opposition from powerful conservative southern Democrats and their ideological counterparts among the Republicans—was until 1965 sufficient to defeat every attempt at universal coverage, whether for all Americans or just those over age 65.

The fight over Medicare illustrates the conditions required for successful reform, even partial reform. Before 1965 the conservative coalition remained formidable. Then the Democratic landslide of 1964 swept away the key institutional bases of conservative power: dilatory tactics symbolically represented by the Rules Committee, control of other key committees without threat from the Democratic caucus, and an ideological balance in the Congress as a whole less liberal than Presidents Kennedy and Johnson. The massive electoral shift of 1964 held a lesson for future reformers. One sufficient condition for reform was the existence of a two-to-one Democratic majority in the House of Representatives, a margin large enough to contain within it an issue majority on Medicare. In retrospect, Medicare might well have emerged from the narrow defeats of the early 1960s; the election of 1964 prevented our knowing.

The Nixon Years: Seeming Consensus, Undeniable Disappointment

By 1970 the topic of national health politics had shifted from Medicare back to national health insurance. Although it is difficult for many to remember, the striking feature of the 1970–1974 period was the competition among proponents of different forms of universal health insurance: the catastrophic proposal advocated by Senators Long and Ribicoff, the Kennedy-Corman bill that so closely followed Canada's national operational program of 1971, and the Nixon administration's plan for mandated health insurance for employed Americans (known then as the Comprehensive Health Insurance Plan, or CHIP).

The lesson of this period is surely relevant today. Reform failed because shifting coalitions defeated every attempt at compromise. The majority that agreed on reform consisted of factions committed to different proposals. The more modest reforms—such as the Long-Ribicoff bill—seemed *too* modest to those who wanted to translate the negative consensus into universal, broad coverage. The proposal for employer-mandated insurance—what President Clinton in fact would later propose—seemed indirect, incomplete, and incapable of cost control to those favoring more straightforward forms of national health insurance. And even Senator Edward Kennedy, who moved from the more ambitious version of national health insurance to a compromise plan that he and the powerful Representative Wilbur Mills (D. Ark.) could accept, was incapable of generating majority support among a coalition of liberal and conservative Democrats.

It is no wonder that so many congressional figures from that period are anxious to act this time. The caution here may well be that the lessons of the 1970s are multiple, not simple. What might well have made sense then—namely, mandated, employment-based coverage—need not define the limit of what is possible twenty years later. Indeed, figuring out the impact of twenty years of frustration with partial reform is the major task facing reformers today.

The Contemporary Task: Daunting But Doable?

The lessons of history are never simple. What worked once may not, in changed circumstances, work again. What failed may succeed. But some constants in American politics are always relevant.

First, compulsory health insurance, whatever the details, is an ideologically controversial matter that involves enormous financial and professional stakes. Such legislation does not emerge quietly or with broad bipartisan support. Legislative success requires active presidential leadership, the commitment of an administration's political capital, and the exercise of many varieties of persuasion and arm twisting. This FDR was unwilling to do in the New Deal and Richard Nixon refrained from doing in the early 1970s. President Johnson was fully willing to use his legendary legislative energy in 1965, but the composition of the Congress then made it virtually unnecessary to do so. The Medicare bill (H.R. 1 and S. 1 were the numerical symbols) was the focus of the legislative campaign in the first year of his new administration.

Second, the limits of political feasibility are far less distinct than the beltway commentators are likely to recognize. The Johnson administration, anxious to make sure that its first step would be overwhelmingly acceptable, requested only hospital benefits under Medicare. But the oddest thing happened. A combination of liberals anxious to make the Medicare program broader, and conservative Democrats wishing to head off step-by-step expansion later, produced a wider reform than LBJ had requested. Not only was physician insurance (what we know as Part B of Medicare) added by the Ways and Means Committee, but Medicare emerged as part of an unexpected "three-layer cake." No one should assume that a substantive and ideological package sent to the Congress is fixed in stone.

Third, the role of language and emotive symbols in this policy world cannot be overestimated. How the President reaches out to the public, what counts in the evening news and the morning newspapers as the central reform themes, and whether the Congress faces a determined grass-roots movement—all shape the legislative outcome and, even more important, whether the result is sufficiently coherent and implementable to satisfy the expectations for reform. Pressure groups that can prevail in quiet politics are far weaker in contexts of mass attention, as the American Medical Association learned to its regret in the Medicare battle of 1965.

The central lesson of the past—of both defeats and victories such as Medicare—is cautionary in a different sense, however. It is wise to wait if what is acceptable is not workable. It is foolish to hesitate if what is workable can be made acceptable. If the central elements of a workable plan are acceptable, the pace of implementation can be staggered. American political history shows that the opportunities for substantial reform are few and far between, precious enough to make squandering close to a sin.

MAKING SENSE OF THE NATIONAL REFORM DEBATE: LABELS, IDEAS, AND PROPOSALS

The warring camps of medical care reformers and their distinguishing labels had become familiar elements of media coverage by 1993.[6] Terms such as "single-payer" or "managed competition" served as shorthand for complex arguments and ideas. They brought together groups of seemingly like-minded reformers, and they made the debate easier for journalists to cover and, at least in theory, for the public to follow. By now, however, the labels block rather than enhance public understanding and make reform more rather than less difficult to achieve.

If such labels were ever helpful, they are no longer. Labels mask differences within categories of reform (between, for example, different plans called "managed competition") and obscure similarities across categories. It is increasingly clear that the Clinton reform proposal—and any other that could command majority approval in the public or the Congress—will draw on understandings, and incorporate elements, from a variety of reform plans. To foreshadow one of our reform debate suggestions: judge a plan not by its label, but by its provisions, its answers to the basic questions of who should receive what insurance on what terms, financed how, implemented by whom. What is needed and likely—as a matter of substantive as well as political wisdom—is a fusion plan.

Why are the existing approaches to reform (and their labels) so inadequate? Before the positive case can be made for the principles of an acceptable fusion plan, there must be less confusion. To those Americans not immersed in the arcana of medical care reform—which is to say almost everybody, including most journalists—the catch phrases of the health insurance debate must be bewilderingly cryptic. Did any voter, for example, understand President Bush's attack in the spring of 1992 on Bill Clinton's supposed support for a "play-or-pay" plan or of then Governor Clinton's equally earnest denials that his medical reform proposal fell into that category? Less than a year after that 1992 debate, almost no one can remember the heated exchange. And this fact itself indicates how little the public commentary has engaged deeply felt concerns about what would and would not satisfy the widespread yearning for improvement in the financing and (for some) the access to and quality of American medicine.

The labels that ought to be discarded—the lingo of intense scrutiny since at least the late 1980s—what do they mean? What are the appropriate connections between a descriptive label and the guiding ideas about medical reform it is meant to express? How are both linked to the details of particular reform proposals, anyway?

In the language of reformers, a *single-payer* plan is one in which health insurance is paid for by government, out of funds it collects from individuals (and, possibly, employers). Many of the proposals typically sorted into this category are modeled on Canada's universal health insurance, a program administered by the ten provinces which manages to insure all Canadians for all "ordinary and necessary" medical care while spending about 30 percent less per capita than we do. This model, first advanced in American politics in the early 1970s, has been through a cycle of advocacy and attack, submersion and reappearance. By 1993 the leading advocates in the Congress were Senator Paul Wellstone (D., Minn.) and Congressman James McDermott (D., Wash.). The smaller insurance firms—now represented by the Health Insurance Association of America (HIAA)—stand to lose the most from this reform and have acted accordingly, joined by the American Medical Association and a number of other groups. Members of organized labor, especially in rust-belt industries like steel and automobiles, were among the most vocal advocates of single-payer reforms, joined by organizations such as Citizen Action, the magazine *Consumer Reports,* and splinter medical groups such as Physicians for a National Health Plan (PNHP).

Yet many so-called single-payer plans actually involve more than 50 payers, because they call for each state to operate its own disbursement operation. "Single-payer" need not mean one plan for an entire country; it refers to one health insurance organization within a political jurisdiction, which is the central idea (often characterized, however, as too radical for the United States).

The single-payer label, however, tells nothing about how health coverage would be financed under any particular insurance plan, what range of medical benefits would be included, how costs would be controlled within the plan's budget, and other matters far too important to be considered mere details. The label itself inadequately describes both the characteristics of the concrete model to which it refers (Canada's program, for instance) and the core ideas that justify trying to put such a model into operation.

Play-or-pay has been an even less satisfactory moniker. It is used to tag proposals in which employers would be required either to purchase health insurance for their employees and their families (the play option) or to enroll them in a public health insurance program and pay a payroll tax toward the cost (the pay option). But plans that include this mechanism for financing insurance can be considerably more different than they are alike. The financing mechanism, as with the single-payer example, is an utterly incomplete description. For example, some play-or-pay plans would guarantee health insurance for the unemployed as well as for those in the workplace; others would not. (The question here is how universal should a plan be, an issue every proposal must answer.) Some play-or-pay variants would control medical costs through a combination of national and state spending targets as well as hospital rate setting and physician fee schedules; others would not. Calling plans so different by the same name is about as sensible as saying that any car with an automatic transmission must be, ipso facto, a Ford.

The third label, *managed competition,* had a much shorter shelf life than seemed imaginable at the outset of the Clinton presidency. The expression was so much in vogue after Clinton's use of the tag late in the presidential campaign that one speaker at a January 1993 retreat for congressional staff members said, "I don't know what we're going to do, but whatever it is, we'll call it managed competition."

Such a cynical embrace of labels—as if they need have no direct connection to substance—is hardly surprising in American politics. Recent experience provides many examples; the much-touted welfare reform legislation of 1988 (the Family Support Act), for example, experienced such a disappointing gap between aspiration and results that we are again addressing the "reform of welfare" as America "knows it." But ultimately disappointing cynicism is especially regrettable where the reform in question involves the country's largest industry, representing one out of every seven cents of American income.

By April of 1993, however, President Clinton's advisers had drawn back from the "managed competition" tag. According to the *New York Times,* the health task force officials who briefed the press "ridiculed" the very expression "managed competition."[7] They tried to distance themselves from those idea promoters who had most forcefully insisted that competition among health insurance plans—not budget limits on how much money was available to medical care—was the core element in workable cost control. Where once "managed competition" and "health insurance purchasing cooperatives (HIPCs)" were the rage, the evident effort was to substitute "health security" and "health alliances" as the defining labels of the President's proposal.

What ideas were associated with the President's earlier embrace of "managed competition"? One central idea is relatively clear: the vision of a restructured medical world in which potential patients ("consumers," in the marketplace lingo) would be organized into purchasing consortia for health insurance, and medical care providers would ideally practice in groups, much like health maintenance organizations (HMOs). Associations of providers would compete for business from the consortia—and the consortia, represented by savvy purchasing agents, would use their buying power (and more and better information about the quality of care from local providers) to try to get good deals for their members.

A lot of suits can go with that tie, however. Proposals that include, or are organized around, the core conception of managed care and regulated competition differ radically from one another. For example, some plans would force doctors into group practices and consumers into buying consortia; others would give doctors and patients the choice of opting out, but would use tax incentives to lure them in. Some proposals would control the fees charged for services patients used outside the "capitated" plans, those paid for on a per capita basis. Others would not, on the assumption that fee-for-service medicine would, like old soldiers, simply fade away if unable to compete on price with prepaid provider groups. Some managed competition plans would phase in universal coverage;[8] others, such as the one proposed by Tennessee Congressman Jim Cooper of the Conservative Democratic Forum in the House of Representatives, would not. And some would put all of American medical care under expenditure targets; others—by now you will have seen the pattern—would not.

There is another contention in our argument that may already have

struck readers: these ostensibly different models of reform can have, at
least in some of their variants, a great deal in common. For instance,
the public organization that purchases coverage for the uninsured and
the employees of some businesses in a play-or-pay plan looks and
functions a lot like the purchasing consortium in the plan currently
favored by the Clinton administration. Both, moreover, look and function a lot like a state board in the state-by-state version of a single-
payer plan. The three reform archetypes, moreover, are by no means
mutually exclusive. Why can't a plan include universal coverage to a
standard set of benefits (as in most single-payer proposals), build around
a base of employer-financed coverage (as the play-or-pay strategy envisioned), *and* encourage the reform of medical care purchasing and
provision (as the managed competition strategy suggests)?

The answer is that it can. Whether the American public will understand that possibility depends in part on how disciplined a debate we
have over the President's proposal in 1994 and beyond. Useful debate
requires not only discipline, but breadth of information. We have not
had sustained attention to a wide range of reform possibilities. From
time to time attention has concentrated on international models (particularly Canada and Germany). But the pattern has been one of initial
enthusiasm, largely mindless criticism, and then neglect. Likewise,
within the United States there are so-called all-payer proposals (as in
New York) that have gotten little national attention. As a result, the
alternatives have narrowed to modest incremental steps versus wholesale transformations of both the financing and the delivery of American
medical care. It is for these reasons that scholarship directed at understanding medical care reform is now so important.

Substituting programmatic fusion for policy confusion is surely called
for. What is needed is not a new paradigm, but no paradigm—an eclectic
approach to medical reform that puts much more emphasis on what
works than on what we call it. But on what principles would a fusion
plan be constructed? After all, without guiding central principles the
appeal to fusion is no improvement over the very label-mongering we
have criticized.

GUIDELINES FOR REFORM AND DEBATE

Sensible reform should build on three fundamental principles.
First, the three elements of the medical crisis—cost, access, and quality—are interconnected. We cannot solve one problem without attending to the other two. If we put all our emphasis on controlling health

spending, quality and access may well suffer. If we focus solely on making sure that everybody has health insurance coverage, cost will rise and quality may erode. And if we do nothing but improve the (highly variable) quality of American medical care, fewer and fewer people will have access to more and more expensive services.

Second, we need reform that can work quickly—that would clamp down on cost increases, cover the more than 37 million uninsured, and lay the groundwork for improvements in quality sooner rather than later. With medical spending increasing at nearly twice the rate of general inflation, tens of millions of Americans risk life without health insurance, and with so many suffering needlessly we ought to be impatient. The longer we wait to fix the medical care system, the harder the job will be.

Third, we need to be prudent. The stakes are too high—in terms of health, psychological security, and financial cost—to put all our faith in one theory or model or mechanism. We should build, to the extent we can, a plan that minimizes failure in the course of seeking success. It should be a reform plan that is, to borrow a term from the computer industry, fault tolerant.

The development of a fusion plan is in some respects easier than it appears, in part because so much of the work has already been done. Many of the reform proposals advanced in recent years (and tagged with one of the three standard-issue labels) are, much more than is commonly acknowledged, admixtures of elements from the "pure" categories. The point applies, for instance, to the plan spelled out in September 1992 by candidate Clinton—one that he (and numerous commentators) described then as a managed competition strategy, but that was in fact something of a hybrid. And the Clinton administration's 1993 proposal is a hybrid as well.

ACCEPTABLE REFORM: FROM PRINCIPLES
TO CHARACTERISTICS

The basic characteristics of a fusion plan—one with both substantive and political merit—are literally strewn about, awaiting assemblage. They include:

1. Financing. What is required is broad-based financing— spreading the costs of medical care, not concentrating them as we do now on the old, the low-income group, or those without employment-based coverage. Small firms and

those with individual policies face premiums far higher
than those large groups pay. Compulsory employer-based
financing is one possible reform, but whenever the government mandates payment, there is a corresponding public
responsibility to limit the burden on any particular group.
And how tying health insurance to employment compli-
cates work force mobility is an issue that must be addressed.

2. Universal eligibility and broad coverage. No one should be
   without insurance protection against the costs of illness,
   injury, and disease. Beyond that, health insurance should
   cover what Americans regard as "ordinary and necessary"
   medical care. Benefits should be free of the obfuscation,
   nasty surprises, and exclusions patients and medical care
   professionals regard as senseless. The core of this commitment is clear: acute and chronic illness, preventive care,
   visits to doctors, prescription drugs. The periphery is necessarily less certain, but, in my judgment, benefits should
   extend to the care of the chronically mentally ill, substance
   abusers, and the frail. These services require special constraints and attention, since they are particularly subject to
   uncontrollable expansion.

3. Tough cost controls that would keep spending in bounds.
   We need to limit medical budgets to the nation's rate of
   growth, not to multiples of that rate. There are many details here that may vary, but the options supported by international experience all include a prospective budget
   limit on affordable outlays. Budget limits, of course, make
   explicit the rationing (allocation) of care, whereas market
   competition masks it.

4. Rewards for the creation of more efficient groups of providers, who are responsive to patients within the discipline
   of limited budgets. Accurate information about medical
   performance would reward those groups whose practices
   are exemplary but not well known. Reductions in the tax
   deductibility of employer contributions to expensive plans
   would help more efficient providers and insurers.

5. Measures to simplify health insurance for patients, payers,
   and providers. These include a standard set of benefits, a
   single claim form (instead of the thousands of different
   forms now bedeviling us), and electronic billing. (Experts

estimate that as much as 20 percent of what Americans spend on medical care goes to pay for administration and paperwork. That amounted to an estimated $180 billion in 1993.) Simplification alone ought to save tens of billions of dollars, let alone the nonfinancial costs of contemporary complexity, confusion, and uncertainty.

6. Institutions of clear accountability for the cost, quality, and accessibility of the care provided. Better information about the quality of care is needed so as to reduce the amount of unnecessary or inappropriate treatment (including increased research on the effects of alternative procedures, and data that enable patients and their doctors to judge the quality of care offered by providers and provider groups). The essential feature, however, is knowing who is to be held to account for performance, a requirement that may well take varying forms in the diverse settings of American states. Explicit attention must be paid to monitoring the quality of care to groups that are especially vulnerable (the chronically ill) or especially hard to represent (the poor and the scattered).

7. Freedom of choice. No reform that ignores professional concerns about autonomy will prove workable. But autonomy need not extend to charging whatever one wishes. No reform that limits patients' choice of doctor is desirable when dictated by financial pressures falling disproportionately on less affluent or more sickly Americans. Where choice is constrained—whether by explicit benefit limits or by restrictions on the supply of providers or facilities— American politics produces hyperbolic talk about "regulation" and "rationing." Most of that talk ignores the extent to which choices are already constrained by the widespread dispersion of managed care in American medicine.

8. Means of consultation and redress. Measures that regularly and transparently express patient and provider concerns, within budget constraints, are essential. This feature is linked to the mechanisms of accountability, but raises separable issues. For example, Americans have little experience in formal negotiation among parties interested in the benefits and burdens of public programs. The American penchant for disinterested umpires to resolve clashes of interest makes it difficult to legitimate straightforward bar-

gaining structures. We lack Europe's vital institutions of
corporatism, the participation of those who will be affected
by public policy in the working out of means to settled
ends and of feeding back information about performance,
glitches, and needless conflict.

None of this discussion of what constitutes sensible reform standards
presumes that the refinement of a reform program, the development of
political support for it, and its implementation will be easy. But the
alternative to fusion—protracted squabbling among rival factions—is
undoubtedly less appealing.[9]

Part I

Medical Care Politics:
Constraints on Reform

Chapter 2
How We Got to Where We Are:
American Health Care Politics,
1970 to 1990

The history of medicine in the United States from 1970 to 1990 was marked by troubled change.[1] Senator Edward Kennedy's 1972 book, *In Critical Condition: The Crisis in America's Health Care*,[2] reflected in its title an atmosphere of urgency in the early 1970s. Indeed, this sense of trouble was so widespread that Republicans and Democrats, liberals and conservatives competed over which form of national health insurance to offer in response. In 1974, for instance, the now-forgotten Kennedy-Mills proposal received extended consideration in the finance committees of the Congress, as did the Nixon CHIP plan and the catastrophic health insurance bill of Senators Long and Ribicoff. It all seems very long ago, looking back from the post-Reagan era, this earlier flurry of proposals and stalemate over universal government health insurance.[3]

In the 1990s the picture is very different, politically and intellectually. Very few figures of political significance confidently promote government-financed universal health insurance, for the nation or for a partic-

From *Quarterly Review of Economics and Business*, Vol. 30, No. 4 (Winter 1990), pp. 32–42. Copyright © The Trustees of the University of Illinois. Reprinted by permission.

The support of the Russell Sage Foundation for a fellowship year (1987–1988) during which this article was written is gratefully acknowledged.

ular state. The deficits of the Reagan and Bush years continue to dominate political discourse and set severe limits on what seems sensible to discuss. Intellectually, we are living with the debris of the reform mentality of the 1970s and 1980s—a mentality that turned first to bureaucratic realignments as a means for rationalizing medical care provisions and then, when those strategies seemed to fail, emphasized competition and privatization in a single-minded preoccupation with cost control.

REGULATORY PROMISES AND FAILURE

The forms of governmental realignment that were chosen to "rationalize" medical care, although each alone certain to disappoint, collectively were regarded as incremental steps toward more sensible governmental intervention in the financing of health services. The regulation that in fact emerged was dispersed bureaucratically, disconnected from the major financing of care, and celebrated with visions of eventual success no reasonable analyst should have accepted. Health planning emerged in 1974—205 little agencies all over the country, equipped with the authority to say no to major capital expansion but lacking the financial carrot to induce anyone to move in a different direction. Professional Standards Review Organizations (PSROs)—established by the federal government to monitor quality of care—were relegated in 1972 to a different set of agencies, dominated by physicians and disconnected in practice from the payment systems of Medicare, Medicaid, or commercial and nonprofit health insurance plans. Medicare and Medicaid, once separate organizationally, were technically joined in what is now known as the Health Care Financing Administration (HCFA) of the Department of Health and Human Services. But this new agency failed to unify Medicare and Medicaid administration, much less have an impact on health planning.

All through the 1970s observers complained about the uneven distribution of care and the relatively high rates of inflation in medicine, but, as with the weather according to Mark Twain, little was altered. The Carter administration supported serious legislation to contain hospital costs but was defeated in both 1978 and 1979 by a combination of hospital opposition, distrust of Carter's team, and more general skepticism about whether the federal government could accomplish what it promised. Inflation continued unabated amid rhetoric about a "voluntary effort" to control costs by the health industry and the emergence of a new set of actors who came to play much more important roles in American medicine.

COMPETITION AS AN ANSWER

Attracted by the gold mine of funds flowing through a system of retrospective, cost-based reimbursement, the captains of American capitalism came to see opportunity where the politicians had found causes for complaint. In the hospital world itself, small chains of for-profit hospitals—the Humanas and Hospital Corporations of America, to name the most prominent examples concentrated in the South—grew into large companies throughout the disappointing regulatory decade of the 1970s. The growth of Health Maintenance Organizations (HMOs)—slower than promised by the enthusiasts of the 1973 legislation—came to include for-profit firms as well. Industrial giants like Baxter-Travenol and American Hospital Supply took their conventional dreams of competitive growth and extended them to vertical and horizontal integration.[4] A glut of physicians started to come into practice, weakening the traditional power of doctors to determine their terms of work.

All of these changes in the structure of American medicine took place within the context of increasingly antiregulatory and anti-Washington rhetoric. Democrats and Republicans alike had been influenced by a generation of academic policy analysts—mostly economists—who ridiculed the costliness and captured quality of the decisions taken by supposedly independent regulatory agencies in Washington. The Civil Aeronautics Board and the airlines industry came to represent the distortions likely when government regulates industry and, with time, the convention of describing any set of related activities with economic significance as an "industry" demythologized medicine as well. So, even before the Reagan administration came into office, the time was ripe for celebrating "competition" in medicine, getting government off the industry's back, and letting the fresh air of deregulation solve the problems of access, cost, and quality.

The irony is that the most consequential health initiative of the 1980s—Medicare's prospective payment system by diagnosis-related groups (DRGs)—was an exceedingly sophisticated, highly regulatory form of administered prices that changed the incentives offered hospitals. And, what was more, the federal deficit made unthinkable a direct attack on the problem of 30 to 40 million Americans who lack anything resembling decent health insurance.

So, more than 20 years after talk of a medical world in critical

Table 2.1
Popular support for national health insurance (percent of those polled)

View	Aug. 1978	Nov. 1978	July 1979
Favor	64	61	61
Oppose	31	33	31
No view	5	6	7

Source: Robert Y. Shapiro and John T. Young, "The Polls: Medical Care in the United States," *Public Opinion Quarterly,* Vol. 50 (1986), p. 423.

condition, we have made little progress in the search for a cure. The problems of access have worsened as we continue to add to the list of the uninsured and the underinsured. The relative rate of medical inflation continues its relentless rise and shows no signs of slowing, and truly extraordinary changes in the rules of the professional game are taking place as American capitalism flexes its muscles on the $650 billion industry we used to call medicine.

COMPETITION VERSUS REGULATION: THE NATURE OF THE DEBATE

At one extreme in the debate over public health expenditures is the idea of complete government control over and administration of medical care. Some Americans—policymakers and medical care professionals as well as ordinary citizens—think that the only way to get the problems of America's health care system under control is to follow the model of the British National Health Service.[5] That model, however, invokes the unhappy image of rationing of care and long waits for all but the most pressing medical problems. It also conjures up images of "socialized" medicine, with all the loss of individual control and freedom of choice for both practitioner and patient that that slogan implies. The widely acknowledged seriousness of American medicine's present problems does not mean that there is clear public support for either the British policy or even for a version of national health *insurance* modeled on the Canadian plan. (See, however, the discussion of the American public's opinion about health and medical care later in this chapter and in Tables 2.1 and 2.2.)

At the other extreme in American health policy debates in the early 1980s was a set of ideas known as the "competitive health strategy."[6] Though their arguments vary, advocates of competition believe that

Table 2.2
Popular opinion on the American health system (percent of those polled)

View	1982	1983	1984
On the whole, the health care system works pretty well; only minor changes are necessary to make it work better.	19	21	26
There are some good things in our health system, but fundamental changes are needed to make it work better.	47	50	49
The American health care system has so much wrong with it that we need to rebuild it completely.	28	25	21

Source: Shapiro and Young, "The Polls," p. 425.

restructuring the incentives is crucial to the restraint of medical inflation and thus to the control of both public and private health expenditures. Their central policy prescription is the introduction of greater price competition in the delivery of care. In the presence of widespread health insurance, the scope for price competition in premiums is greater than in fees and charges through substantially increased consumer cost-sharing. The striking feature of this perspective is the gap between the rhetoric of competition and the reality of constraints on room to maneuver. An important impediment to the enactment of procompetitive legislation is the indirect connection between effective competitive markets and reductions in medical care expenditures. A competitive strategy, even if implemented, does not produce visible gains in the short run. Even its most optimistic supporters concede that it would take 10 to 15 years for a competitive market to develop and, if effective, to begin to reduce medical expenditures in any given area. During a development period, medical care outlays would continue to increase, as they in fact did during the 1980s, and to put pressure on politicians to "do something."

The eventual outcome of a competitive strategy is uncertain, since it has not been implemented on a wide scale anywhere in the postwar period. For all these reasons, the reality of health politics in the 1980s was one of incremental steps of both a regulatory and a competitive variety, what one might call "agitated incrementalism."[7] There is little coherent public concern about the rising costs of health care in the United States, though polls that are discussed later do reveal continuing public anxiety. The concerns that matter are about the cost of care to individuals (in premiums or cost-sharing when ill), to firms (in increased expenditures for employee health insurance), and to governments (in rising outlays for particular programs—Medicare quite obviously for federal officials, Medicaid for state and federal officials). Worry about relative inflation in medical care—the concern that the society is spending more for care in the aggregate than its citizens receive in benefits— is an academic's problem. America may well be, as Brian Abel-Smith wrote some years ago, a country where we receive insufficient "value for money;"[8] but where health is concerned, the public worries more about access and quality than about value for money.

As a result, cost containment, when seriously attempted, arises from actions to control the rising costs of medical care to particular payers, most prominently the federal government and hardly less so to particular states and corporations.[9] The problems with that approach are all related to the obvious fact that actions that save federal (or state or corporate) dollars do not necessarily constitute anti-inflationary successes. Indeed, federal actions and policies have substantially shifted costs from the national government to other payers and have had little or no effect on total health care expenditures.

Equally worrisome, reduced federal outlays may have resulted from the denial of care—hardly a story of Medicare's beneficiaries receiving similar services at lower cost, or more services at the same price per unit, or more health results at given price. Budget deficit reduction, in short, is a goal that can be reached by a variety of means, only some of which meet acceptable criteria for national health policy. Nor is the cost shifting of other particular payers in America's pluralistic arena of health care finance any more acceptable as a national health policy.

The United States has no consensus regarding either the character of the problem of rising medical costs or its possible solution.[10] As Ken Wing has acutely noted, there is a "divisive political struggle among interest groups [in which] defining the nature of the problem is as much in controversy as is fashioning a remedy; and [in which] the reform or remedy sought for one problem . . . would only exacerbate the problems of the others."[11]

This is as accurate a description of these two decades of health politics as I know. "The reasons for this political state of affairs," Wing readily admits, "are not altogether clear."[12] It is quite true that the delivery of medical care "can be simultaneously described as a system on the brink of crisis and as a strong and growing industry, with seeming equal accuracy."[13] In attempting to explain this situation, one needs first to emphasize the enormous influence of providers in the imbalanced political marketplace of health policy. And, worsening that imbalance is the lack of sustained public opinion marshaled around any one of the various formulations of the problems of cost, access, and quality of American medicine. Surely a very large measure of the explanation for our health circumstances is the pluralism of American politics and the parallel dispersion of countervailing power in both the political and economic marketplaces. Our federalism has spread the authority for regulating medical care between the national government and the many states. Our financing splits private and public payers, with considerable discrepancies among these in each sector.

Two explanatory factors for the cost crisis in American medicine, then, become central. Medical care is a merit good, widely insured through work, a part of the private and public welfare state we have fashioned in America. The fragmentation of finance has meant that, once payers are aroused, the problem they separately address is that of their own costs, not of American medicine. Pluralistic finance, combined with extensive third-party coverage, is a predictable recipe for inflation. Only those regimes that have concentrated the stakes of medical payers—Great Britain, Canada, France, for instance—have been able to restrain the forces of medical inflation. And such countervailing power is but the necessary condition for restraint; political will is also essential. In some cases, as in Sweden, the stakeholders with concentrated authority have *chosen* to spend more on medical care. But they have made such choices through balancing the gains and losses of expenditures. In the United States, we have *discovered* our inflating health outlays, not chosen them.

REACTIONS TO ELI GINZBERG'S "LOOKING BACK, LOOKING AHEAD"

Professor Ginzberg's paper which appeared in 1990 in the *Quarterly Review of Economics and Business,* presents some obvious difficulties and opportunities for the commentator. I have elsewhere reviewed Ginzberg's book-length treatment of this topic.[14] Extensive discussion of each of his many contentions would, therefore, be redundant as well as tedious. Moreover, Ginzberg fetchingly entitles his contribution; he has more years than most analysts to look back on and, from the evidence of his vigor, quite a number to look ahead to. An experienced and prolific interpreter of America's health circumstances, Ginzberg writes with a clarity that makes plain what he means.

This is, of course, welcome to the commentator. I find much to agree with and much to disagree with in this pithy essay.

The area of agreement should be obvious from the foregoing discussion of medical inflation and the political difficulties in addressing it within the present American context. What I have labeled the "imbalanced medical market" in America[15] is elaborated in the Ginzberg discussion. His skepticism about particular fads in cost control—Preferred Provider Organizations (PPOs), HMOs, utilization review, and "similar approaches in which financial risk and incentives are shared with providers"—seem to me wise and ignored at our peril. Professor Ginzberg is anything but shy in making his forecasts, but it is very difficult for me, in such agreement here, to find serious fault in them. The dismal scientists in health cost containment are not, as conventionally understood, the economists. They are the political scientists, generally speaking, and here Ginzberg joins intellectually with Harvey Sapolsky, Larry Brown, James Morone, myself, and others in political science to cast great doubt on the relentless dreaminess of a cost-contained, competitive world of medicine. (Incidentally, this judgment is shared by another distinguished health economist, Robert G. Evans of the University of British Columbia, whose landmark book, *Strained Mercy,* is admired by Ginzberg and ignored by most other American health economists.)[16]

There is agreement between the economist Ginzberg and the great bulk of political analysts of medicine about the problem of medical care costs. It is an instance of common judgment about a topic conventionally monopolized by economists. It is when Ginzberg turns to subjects of public opinion and the sources of American public policy that he ventures into the zone of political science and, I must say, wanders very far afield. Let me illustrate with two examples.

The area of disagreement arises from Ginzberg's misreading of the state of American public opinion about medicine in the postwar period, particularly the character and level of support for governmental health insurance. His overall judgment is that American health politics, like much else, changes incrementally, with "periodic crises." With this, I and most other political analysts would have little quarrel. But he moves from the descriptive view of incrementalism to its normative version with Panglossian ease. We are told that "there is no evidence that the American people want to change [the] system" of medical care they had in the 1980s. The same goes retrospectively for the immediate postwar period; few really wanted national health insurance, according to Ginzberg. Indeed, he claims "the fact that only a small part of the voting public favored NHI . . . has not been widely appreciated." And, if evidence about the beginning of the period and the end are not enough, we are assured that "the general satisfaction of the U.S. public health with the prevailing system of private insurance" explains why the national health insurance aspirations of Jimmy Carter led nowhere.

The difficulties with this formulation are not that they are implausible, but that they are simply wrong. And they are presented with a cavalier disregard of the published literature that is simply staggering. One of the benefits of long study is a sure sense of one's own views; one of its liabilities is an easily acquired disinclination to investigate further what one assumes to be true. In the case of public opinion, the findings of recent scholarship demolish the portrait of complacency presented in this sketch.

It is simply not the case that a minority of Americans favored national health insurance immediately after World War II. But, leaving that historical period for the moment, the 1970s were not an instance where the undeniable failure of national health insurance legislation expressed the lack of popular support. An NBC poll during the Carter years shows precisely that. In answer to the question, "Do you favor or oppose a national program of health insurance giving medical and hospital care to everyone, with the government paying part of the cost?", as Table 2.1 shows, the response was consistently favorable in 1978–1979.

Nor were the 1978–1979 findings restricted to that one-year period. The *New York Times*/CBS polling between 1976 and 1981 showed majorities of those with opinions "in favor . . . of national health insurance, financed by tax money, and paying for most forms of care."[17] And, if that is not enough to suggest how inaccurate the Ginzberg portrait is of American public opinion, consider the Harris polls of the early 1980s probing how satisfied Americans were with the state of our medical care. Respondents were asked to report "which of the following statements [came] closest in expressing [their] overall view of the American health care system." The results are shown as Table 2.2 for the 1982–1984 period.

More than 70 percent of these Americans—the sum of the lower rows in the table—agreed that American medicine needed either fundamental change or complete rebuilding. This is not a credible basis for anyone to claim that Americans were satisfied with their medical system in the first half of the 1980s. And since these data are not remarkable for the period 1970–1988, Ginzberg's assertions about public opinion are, in the technical sense, incredible.[18]

It is worth asking, in closing, how such an experienced observer of American medical arrangements as Eli Ginzberg could have been so wrong on this point. Part of the reason, of course, is that public opinion is a subject on which presumption and practical experience are very uncertain guides. One can sometimes understand institutions with a powerful theory guided by sensible observation. Mancur Olson did so with his remarkable book, *The Logic of Collective Action*.[19] Ginzberg's remarks about the behavior of American hospitals and physicians include many such compelling judgments. But he does not know the public opinion literature and, remarkably, seems innocent of the dangers of bold statements of fact that are not substantiated. Yet there may be another process at work. Economists generally begin by assuming that people want what they seek. It is not a large leap to conclude that, if behavior persists, in this case the continuing growth of demand for American medical care, consumers get what they sought and wanted. This is not very different from the Panglossian view that we have the best of all possible worlds. Or, put another way, the evidence that one likes what one has is that one has it and does not revolt. When we have independent measures of opinion, this intellectual leapfrogging is simply unwarranted.

The relationships among American opinion, health policies, and national results are no simple matter. To say that we get the system we have wanted, using as evidence the system we have, is faulty reasoning. The results we have represent bargains, outcomes (anticipated and unanticipated), and shifting victories for particular parties—none of them neat and simple. The virtue of Ginzberg's analysis is his clear skepticism about simple panaceas working in this complex area of political economy. His vices emerge when he ventures into subjects where crystallized common sense is no guide to what is the case.

Chapter 3
Medical Care Crises and
the Welfare State

Most policy debates in most countries are parochial affairs. They address national "problems," cite historical and contemporary national developments in a particular domain (e.g., pensions, urban affairs, transportation), and embody conflicting visions of what policies the particular country should adopt. Only rarely are the experiences of other nations seriously considered. When cross-national examples are employed in such parochial struggles, their use is typically part of policy warfare more than of policy understanding.[1]

So it was in the United States during the postwar period that Britain's "socialized medicine" became a familiar epithet in discussions of national health insurance and, later, Medicare. For others, the "advanced" welfare state of Sweden has been a model of how pensions should be structured. In child welfare, the universal child allowances of many European nations have been the exemplary instances—or criticized

This chapter is a slightly revised version of "American Medical Policy and the Crisis of the Welfare State: A Comparative Perspective," *Journal of Health Politics, Policy, and Law*, Vol. 11, No. 4 (1986), Tenth Anniversary Issue. Copyright © 1986 by Duke University. Reprinted by permission.

Support for the research and writing of the paper was provided, in part, by a grant from the Henry J. Kaiser Family Foundation of Menlo Park, California, to T. R. Marmor and the Institution for Social and Policy Studies at Yale University.

symbols—of what family policy should include. Historically, the focus is national and programmatic; cross-nationally, the emphasis is on similar problems or policies abroad. Only very rarely in social policy debates has the agenda included a broad review of other national experiences with a set of related, but distinct, policies. When such review takes place, it more typically occurs in economic policy, where the cross-national treatment of fiscal, monetary, and industrial policy issues is far more developed?[2]

This chapter takes as its focus the connection between medical policy concerns and the postwar development of welfare states in the advanced industrial democracies. First, I discuss the widespread cross-national questioning of the welfare state in the wake of the stagflation of the post-1973 period. For the past two decades, the "crisis" of the welfare state has become a staple of policy discussion in otherwise quite varied regimes. Exactly what is alleged to have occurred? Second, I examine the evidence about what in fact happened during this period—the information crucial to understanding the response of different polities to the common strain of lower growth rates, inflation, increased unemployment, and large welfare state claims on public expenditure. Finally, I explain how the argument about crisis and the facts about adjustment related to American concerns about medical care in the 1980s.

This chapter's agenda is broad and its commentary summary, but its argument is straightforward. Our medical policy disputes have been substantially changed by the fear that our nation cannot afford its present social programs; attention to the broader welfare context is therefore crucial to understanding American medicine and its politics. It is as if our debates have centered on the distribution and character of an area's fires, without much attention to the direction and velocity of the prevailing wind.

THE ALLEGED CRISIS

The claim of crisis in the welfare state that arose in the 1970s and continued to be voiced in the 1980s called for radical restructuring of the set of social programs that emerged in the Great Depression and postwar period. In America, that claim was strongly identified with the election of Ronald Reagan in 1980 and the subsequent attacks on federal social spending. In Europe, it was certainly associated with the triumph and continued political victories of Margaret Thatcher in Great Britain and with shifts to the right in a number of other political regimes.[3]

The claim of the welfare state's crisis had become a cliché of political debate over the preceding 15 years. That claim is, however, quite ambiguous. Contemporary discussions, relying on unclear and often misunderstood terms, provide a clue to the confusion about exactly what the "troubles of the welfare state" were. Were the social policies of the modern state in crisis, or was the state in crisis because desirable welfare commitments overwhelmed fiscal capacity? What exactly was meant by "the welfare state"? Did it refer to the major spending programs of contemporary governments? If so, leaving defense aside, we are talking about pensions, medical care, education, and housing in different mixes in different countries. Or was legitimacy, rather than expenditure, the issue? Measured by popular support, the major spending programs in health and pensions were cross-nationally popular. Was the crisis then one of finding the means to finance crucial and popular commitments? Or did the problem include governmental extension of authority into disputed policy areas such as abortion and busing in the United States, redistribution toward French-speakers in Canada, "guest workers" in Germany and Sweden, and the like? Simply put, there was no agreement about what the topic was.

The impulse to sort out the disagreements is thus understandable. One approach avoids much of the contentiousness by changing the question from an analytical one to a historical one. That is, as Peter Flora and Arnold Heidenheimer write in their introduction to *The Development of Welfare States in Europe and America*,[4] one can easily move from recent troubles to wondering how it is that the conditions of the 1970s emerged. With this approach the development of welfare states becomes the subject, rather than the character, causes, and implications, of contemporary disputes. It may well be that historical understanding of development will illuminate matters, but there is no assurance of this.

Another approach is to assume we know what the crisis is and proceed to ask about its causes and prospects. This alternative was vividly illustrated by the efforts of the Organization for Economic Co-operation and Development (OECD) in the late 1970s and early 1980s. Two years of preparation went into a conference on social policies in 1980. But the book that emerged from the conference—*The Welfare State in Crisis*[5]—showed how little consensus there actually was about the topic. The book proceeds from the assumption that the papers address the prospects for improving a clearly worrisome state of affairs that was similarly understood by all analysts. Instead, the papers move past one another. Some ask why protest emerged in such a mix of welfare states; others address the trade-offs between investment and consumption policies of the modern state; still others concentrate on the values of citizens in modern states with extensive social programs. Neither the developmental approach nor the premature presumption of agreement promises an adequate understanding of the problems of the welfare state. To understand the crisis debate, other starting points are necessary.

The wide body of literature concerning the welfare state falls into three categories. Some analysts regard the welfare state's growth as the main cause of many political troubles. Most often associated with the apocalyptic right, those who espouse this belief focus on restraining the overreaching state and redeveloping the institutions of the market and the hegemony of individual choice.

Others see the modern state's experience with slowed economic growth as the source of strains *for* social welfare programs. In the middle politically, these center incrementalists are preoccupied with the way in which fiscal strain and stagflation required cutbacks. They view the crisis as caused by fiscal strains on welfare state programs rather than as a result of any inherent feature of welfare state institutions. They assume that with the resumption of economic growth the crisis will abate.

A third group stresses the controversies over particular social programs (usually not fiscally important ones) that reach to issues of legitimate governmental purpose. The proponents of this view see the strains on the welfare state as evidence of the contradictions of modern capitalism, and the crisis in the modern welfare state as a portent of future troubles along the way.

There are, of course, overlaps among these three approaches, and the first two can, without heroic effort, be tightly linked. But there are differences, and they make a difference in mapping the subject.

Approach 1: From social welfare programs to the state's crisis.   There are two different versions of this approach. Both share the view that social welfare programs played a major role in the poor economic performance of the 1970s. At the theory's simplest level, social programs compete with other budget outlays, preventing the proper balance between investment and consumption. Some critics call this the "bankrupting" of the state; they insist on the importance of budgetary competition and the unfortunate consequences of welfare state expansion.[6] The second form of argument stresses the indirect

Table 3.1
Social expenditures in selected OECD *countries: average annual growth rate of deflated[a] social expenditures,[b] 1960–81 (percent)*

Country	1960–1975	1975–1981
Canada	9.3	3.1
France	7.3[c]	6.2
Germany	7.0	2.4
Italy	7.7	5.1
Japan	12.8	8.4
Norway	10.1	4.6
United Kingdom	5.9	1.8
United States	8.0	3.2

a. Deflated expenditures are defined as public expenditures measured at constant GDP prices.
b. Social expenditures are defined as education, health care, pensions, and unemployment compensation.
c. Excluding education.
Source: Organization for Economic Cooperation and Development, *Social Expenditure: 1960–1981, Problems of Growth and Control* (Paris: OECD, 1985), Table 1, p. 21.

consequences of many social programs for the mobility of capital and labor. This argument gives us something worth pondering. But it is important to notice that the causal arguments very differently interpret the undeniable growth of spending in this sector during the 1960s and early 1970s. The first argument treats spending as the problem. In the second argument, the rigidities are not centrally involved with the largest spending programs, though unemployment insurance is certainly both important and moderately prominent in budget terms.

The striking thing about these criticisms is their familiarity. They represent the oldest thread of objection to the initial development of social programs. Fiscally, the most substantial expansion of public social welfare took place in the 1960s and early 1970s (see Table 3.1). This body of criticism became more widely noted only after stagflation strains spread in the wake of the 1973–1974 oil shock.

It is also worth noting that the worst scenario of the bankruptcy view was discredited almost as soon as it was generated. The major spending

programs of the welfare state did not continue to grow as if uncontrolled
by political authorities. Expansion did not continue automatically in the
midst of fiscal strain; everywhere review took place, although often
without clarification.[7] Finally, it is worth noting that big spenders in the
welfare state did not necessarily have the most serious growth problems
in the 1970s. The simple connection between the size of the public
sector (or social welfare sector) and economic growth problems does
not hold up under comparative scrutiny.[8]

   *Approach 2: From the fiscal crisis of stagflation to welfare state
troubles.*   From this point of view, the problem is that the worldwide
recession of the mid-1970s critically threatened the welfare state. The
combination of lower rates of economic growth, increasing levels of
unemployment, and worrisome levels of investment produced strain for
the programs that grew rapidly in the earlier decade. In the short run,
the welfare state programs appropriately cushioned the effects of recent
recession. But because inflation and unemployment increased outlays
when recession reduced government revenues, the fiscal strain became
quickly apparent.[9] For the longer run, the prospects of unavoidable
pressures in medical care and pensions are evident and are sometimes
used to prod present action through panic mongering.[10] For the United
States, the crucial strains in pensions lie in the twenty-first century,
when the baby-boom generation will be old.[11] There is thus time to
adjust taxes, benefits, and retirement conventions. But it is important
to see the difference between the short-term effects of stagflation and
the structural-demographic prospects for major spending programs over
time. It is difficult to exaggerate the fearfulness of these discussions in
the United States, and thus it is important to consider the range of
reactions to common stresses.

   The relation between welfare state growth and present fiscal strain
has another dimension. During the 1960s, when program expansion took
place under exceedingly favorable economic circumstances, very little
policy discussion considered what would happen under adverse economic conditions. The central ideas of the welfare state were canonized,
not analyzed. There was little discussion about alternative means to
settled ends. And in the United States, where the least consensus about
the original purposes of a welfare state had emerged, rapid growth and
uncertain commitment coincided. It is not surprising, from that point
of view, that welfare state laggards like the United States and Canada
have suffered the most diffuse fearfulness about the future.[12] The rates

of growth of social spending in the 1960s could not, in any event, have been sustained forever. But since they rested on optimistic economic assumptions, the reversal in economic fortunes was all the more startling. It is worth reviewing, as I do below, the management of adjustment to worldwide economic downturns, particularly looking at ways of pursuing central objectives with some flexibility but without fears of programmatic betrayal.

Approach 3: Welfare state strains and governmental legitimacy. The two perspectives just outlined need not attack the fundamental purposes of major social welfare programs. The elimination of want, ignorance, squalor, disease, and idleness are aims that are compatible with either the view that remedial programs have grown too costly for economic health or the view that, with less means, more efficient ways to established ends are required. But a third perspective on the social policy strains of the 1970s and 1980s is in one sense more fundamental. It is the view that welfare state programs include some efforts that are wrong—inappropriate employment of public means even if funds are available or the effects on economic vitality are not worrisome. This is what I mean by criticisms of legitimacy.

The particular items of principled objection vary somewhat from one OECD nation to another, but typically they do not center on the major domestic spending programs we have mentioned. In the United States, Aid to Families with Dependent Children (AFDC), abortion, bilingualism, affirmative action, and school busing have dominated the agenda of the most vitriolic debates.[13] The British counterparts to these controversial but fiscally modest programs are the dole and issues of immigrant workers. Not all critics agree on what the state should forswear. But in general, the claim is that family, custom, and local community should regulate these areas more than governmental decree. In particular, there is serious challenge to politics that emerges from court decisions establishing rights where legislative decision has been hesitant, stalemated, or ambiguous.

The striking fact about AFDC finance, for example, has been its modest role in the overall growth of American social welfare expenditures (see Table 3.2). AFDC's prominence in our debate arises from racial and moral concerns far more than from fiscal ones.[14] And in the frustrating efforts to reform public assistance over the years, sweeping legislative reform has not been achieved. Instead a series of legal and political challenges has, in practice, changed the ways in which some

Table 3.2
Total federal expenditures for selected social programs, 1970–1985 (in billions of constant 1985 dollars)

Program	1970	1975	1980	1985
Social Security (OASDI)[a]	78.3	123.4	153.6	186.4
Medicare	17.9	27.4	44.6	69.6
Unemployment insurance	8.1	24.8	22.1	16.1
AFDC (assistant payments program)[c]	10.9[b]	9.9	9.1	8.6
Supplemental security income (SSI)	—	8.4	7.5	8.7

a. Old age, survivors, and disability insurance.
b. Includes aid to needy aged, blind, and disabled adults, which became SSI in 1974.
c. Since 1974, most outlays in the "assistant payments" category have been for AFDC.
Source: Congressional Research Service, *1986 Budget Perspective: Federal Spending for the Human Resource Programs,* February 1986, pp. 55, 81.

assistance is given—by whom, and to whom. Likewise, school busing policies emerged far more prominently through judicial interpretations of the famous 1954 *Brown* decision of the Supreme Court than through decades of legislative debate and policymaking.

In these cases, the argument is less one of retreat from a widely accepted aim than a challenge to the legitimacy of the aim itself. In other nations, analogous challenges to legitimacy have arisen, but not for the same mix of programs. In Sweden and West Germany, both the treatment of "guest workers" and the structure of public education have prodded fundamental questioning.[15] In Canada, the policies toward French Canadians and bilingualism have prompted widespread objection to governmental authority reaching the redistribution of opportunities to different language groups. My claim is simply that such changes, coincident with the fiscal strains in all OECD welfare states, have confusingly shaped the sense of crisis. The addition of legitimacy concerns to fiscal fears has reduced the degree to which more familiar methods of problem solving seem appropriate to the state's contemporary troubles. How different regimes have treated similar controversies is one subject for cross-national research. Particularly relevant here are studies of broadly similar regimes; the possibility of cross-national learning increases substantially as national differences are, in a sense, "controlled."

WHAT ACTUALLY HAPPENED

The differing views just outlined charge in one way or another that the critical flaws of the welfare state programs and thus of the welfare state itself were part of a general dissatisfaction with the modern institutions of government. These assumptions rest on factual mistakes. Cross-national evidence from the 1970s—a time when government revenues were restrained by stagflation and the burdens on the welfare state increased—supports the notion that the major social spending programs remained quite broadly popular. In the United States the major programs (pensions, medical care, and education) never lacked public or political support. Both public opinion polls and the public reaction to attempted cutbacks by the Reagan administration testified to the popularity of these programs. The most vehement criticism of the welfare state largely concentrated on its more fiscally trivial programs.

It is quite clear, however, that the future of the welfare state in countries with large, settled programs cannot possibly replicate the extraordinary growth in social spending that marks the postwar experience. It is equally clear that the slowed growth of social spending in the 1970s and 1980s was due to the combination of slower economic growth and the overwhelming fact that large, mature programs simply could not continue to grow rapidly without imposing steadily increasing opportunity costs.[16] Further sharp increases in already-large government programs would, for instance, impose additional tax burdens on those at the bottom of the income distribution. The defensible argument for selectivity in program growth and spending arises therefore not from ideological rejection of their earlier purpose but from the reality that these very large, settled programs in pension, health care, and education reduce the margins for continued growth in the future.

Klein and O'Higgins use the OECD data from 1985 on social expenditure trends from 1960 to 1981 to analyze the overall pattern as well as the country-by-country and program-by-program variations.[17] Their analysis yields a number of significant conclusions. First, from 1975 to 1981, all the OECD countries reduced the rate of increase in social spending, but none actually reduced real total social expenditures. They all exhibited the capacity to steer their welfare states to hold down spending increases in response to the adverse economic environment.

Second, the reactions of different countries varied both in the extent to which they reduced spending growth and in the priorities accorded different spending programs.

Over the OECD as a whole, the average annual growth rate of real social spending fell between the periods 1960–1975 and 1975–1981 from 8.4 percent to 4.8 percent. Economic growth during the same time periods fell from 4.6 percent to 2.6 percent. National reductions, however, varied by a factor of eight—from 1.1 percent in France to 8.8 percent in the Netherlands. Klein and O'Higgins speculate that such differences may reflect the degree of maturity reached by different welfare states by the mid-1970s (as reflected in the level of social spending in 1975) or the different degrees of economic difficulty experienced after 1975, as well as different political responses.

Their analysis of the cross-sectional data suggests that the rate of growth of social spending was negatively linked to the 1975 spending share, but positively related to subsequent economic growth rates. Thus the higher a country's level of social spending in 1975, the lower its rate of increase in social spending during 1975–1981; and countries with the highest economic growth rates during 1975–1981 could be expected to experience the highest rate of growth in social spending.[18]

Of particular importance for our purposes, however, are the deviations from this general pattern exhibited by a number of the countries, most notably the United States. Table 3.3 uses the measure of income elasticity of social spending to illustrate national differences in the relationship between the change in growth rates of social spending and the degree of economic strain experienced by individual countries.[19] Four countries—Norway, Canada, Japan, and the United States—show substantial declines in their elasticities between the two periods. In other words, these countries experienced significantly less growth in social spending as compared with their overall economic growth during the period 1975–1981 than they did during the 1960–1975 period. The cases of the United States and Norway are particularly interesting because, despite their very different political traditions, they are two of the strongest overreactors. The result in each case reflects a combination of a lower fall in economic growth than the OECD average (0.2 for both countries, as against the OECD average of 2.0) and a greater fall in social spending growth (4.8 and 5.5 points respectively, against an average of 3.6). These data suggest that national perceptions and definitions of fiscal crisis are as important as economic performance in understanding welfare state policymaking.

Table 3.3
Income elasticity^a of social expenditures in selected OECD countries, 1960–75 and 1975–81^b

Country	1960–1975	1975–1981
Canada	1.8	0.9
France	2.2	2.2
Germany	0.8	0.8
Italy	1.4	1.6
Japan	3.9	1.8
Norway	2.4	1.1
United Kingdom	2.2	1.8
United States	2.4	1.0

a. The ratio of the growth rate of nominal social expenditures to the growth rate of nominal GDP.
b. Or latest year available.
Source: Organization for Economic Cooperation and Development, *Social Expenditure: 1960–1981, Problems of Growth and Control* (Paris: OECD, 1985), Table 1, p. 22.

Klein and O'Higgins also find significant national variations in spending changes by program for the major welfare state programs—health, pensions, and education. Their analysis shows that many more countries reacted to the crisis by restraining spending growth for education and health care rather than by curbing spending for pensions. From 1960 to 1975, spending on health care grew at the fastest rate: in the seven largest OECD economies, real spending grew by an average of 9.0 percent, as compared to 8.2 percent for pensions and 6.2 percent for education. From 1975 to 1981, average annual growth rates for health care and education fell to 3.4 percent and 1.4 percent respectively, while that for pensions only fell to 6.8 percent. Their data suggest that there is some scope—given flexibility and adaptiveness—for accommodating new demands (such as those created by the aging of the population) by holding back the growth rates of other programs and changing public spending priorities.

The experience between 1975 and 1981, as Klein and O'Higgins argue, shows how "a common economic crisis was translated into very

different social spending responses by national political systems." This
calls for an analysis of the impact of politics and policies on welfare
state spending,[20] and raises broad questions about the claim that the
crisis of the welfare state reflected "some systematic affliction common
to all the advanced capitalist countries, independent of national political
ideology or institutions."[21]

AMERICA'S DISTINCTIVE RESPONSE

The comparative evidence above provides the basis for inter-
preting the distinctive American responses to stagflation. By the mid-
1970s, the United States had moved considerably from its postwar
position as the laggard in the scope and financing of social welfare
programs toward being a mature welfare state, with a large, fully in-
dexed (after 1972) pension scheme. Our governmental health insurance
for the poor and the elderly, although not on the universal scale of other
countries, had expanded considerably and contributed to that growth.
We had an apparatus of social welfare programs that covered a wide
range, and the key spending components—old-age pensions and medical
care—were inflating just as in the rest of the world. The predictable
result was fiscal stress as stagflation increased program outlays and as
lowered economic growth reduced governmental revenues. These features were common across the world of industrial democracies. Where
the United States differed was in the more limited degree of acceptance
of the welfare state's purposes and clarity about its aims. The growth
of the early 1970s had largely come from unexpected inflation and
pension indexation, not from a fundamental reexamination of purpose.
The result was that the maturing American welfare state had fewer
means to cushion the strains macroeconomic developments brought. It
was all too easy to confuse economic problems facing the welfare state
with problems within the programs of the American welfare state.

The reasons for this mismatch between scale of effort and national
understanding have much to do with the structure of American politics
and the nature of its typical policy developments. The fragmentation of
American politics puts an enormous premium on consensus, on gaining
agreement so that the multiple veto points of the polity can be avoided.
But agreement on the existence of a problem is far easier to secure than
agreement on an appropriate policy response. The result is that American politics moves by fits and starts, with long periods of gestation and
sudden bursts of political action when issue majorities are assembled.
As long as the question is whether sufficient support exists for taking

action, the political incentives direct reformers to concentrate on problem symptoms and the broad legitimacy of desirable remedies.

So it was that in the long battle over Medicare contending parties debated endlessly whether the medical troubles of America's aged warranted anything like a social insurance response. The debate between 1950 and 1965 centered less on the programmatic details of Medicare proposals than on whether the circumstances and claims of the aged warranted a central government remedy as opposed to a private or a state remedy. The very name of the program—Medicare—misdescribed the limited hospitalization proposals that in fact constituted the legislative agenda in the late 1950s and early 1960s.[22] What the public expected was much broader than what the Medicare legislative battle addressed. And when a broader Medicare program unexpectedly emerged from the bargaining of 1965, there was little public agreement about the program's purposes and the cost-control implications of the program's design. Likewise, the indexation of Social Security in 1972 (the result of congressional bargaining in an election year) produced long-run increases in Social Security payments without a glimmer of broad review.

Programmatic innovation thus proceeded without purposive clarity or agreement on strategies of implementation. The Vietnam War meant that expenditures for "guns" accompanied increases in the "butter" programs of the welfare state. The result was predictable, if lamentable. The United States faced the stagflation strains of the mid-1970s with the worst of all combinations: a large, rapidly growing system of social programs and a very incomplete comprehension of where we were coming from and what we were hoping to accomplish.

From the inability of mature welfare states to continue to grow on the scale of expansion during the first two decades of the postwar period, it follows that altered modes of adjustment were necessary. In making that adjustment it made an enormous difference precisely how the welfare state was conceptualized. For most of the OECD countries, the diagnosis was straightforward: the challenge of welfare state adjustments was to determine how to make modest changes in the large spending programs so as to respond to reduced revenues and to open up opportunity for more targeted initiatives. It was not possible to expand on a number of policy fronts. Yet rather modest tinkering with large spending programs would free up substantial financial resources. In the short run, minor adjustments would relieve financial strain. In the longer run, policy flexibility would emerge from the slow adjustment of details in the shape and administration of the medical care, pension, education, and housing programs that make up the bulk of OECD social expenditures. The implication was clear as well. Time spent worrying about how to make marginal adjustments in major programs made sense because the relative benefit of freeing up resources would be very great when the economic constraints were so serious. Tinkering, for the OECD, was sensible and, in the main, forthcoming.[23]

The adjustments in American politics did not closely follow this model. On the one hand, the financial strain of stagflation did produce marginal changes—the Social Security amendments of 1977 and the more substantial adjustments of 1983 in the wake of the Greenspan Commission. No major new social policy initiative commanded national attention until the Clinton health reform proposals of 1993. In this sense, deficit politics have constrained welfare state development sharply. On the other hand, the adjustments we have made have occasioned fundamental debate and prompted great fearfulness. In that sense, the tinkering that actually emerged brought degrees of social insecurity that the scale of adjustments hardly warrants. Two examples illustrate this process.

In Social Security, fiscal strain evoked fears of bankruptcy. The doomsday scenarios made small adjustments all the more difficult, as partisan opponents traded specters of doom or complacency. Indeed, both a special commission and the most extraordinary use of twenty-first-century forecasts were required to prod the marginal action of the Congress in 1983.[24] In welfare reform, by contrast, the fiscal stakes were far smaller, but there was a similar cycle of crisis mongering and profound questioning. In this instance, no adjustments of public assistance policy were enough to affect the American welfare state's fiscal stability over the long run. Yet the discussion took place without this fiscal fact in clear view.

Both these instances illustrate the mismatch of rhetoric and reality as well as the constraints of deficit politics. Politicians get credit for having addressed the programs for the poor critically or sympathetically. But changes in the programs for poor people are incapable of affecting the fiscal realities of limits on a large welfare state. On the other hand, Social Security and (to a lesser extent) Medicare are precisely where fiscal strain is apparent. Yet our politics express the appeal of these popular programs in the form of limiting adjustments, making Social Security a sacred cow for fear that poachers will attack the whole herd. The result is a social policy debate full of smoke and mirrors, a world of fantasy where the debate departs substantially from the margin of

responsible adjustment—in benefits and taxation—that long-run altera-
tions will require.

IMPLICATIONS FOR MEDICAL CARE

The concern of this chapter is whether the cross-national evidence and the general policy directions illuminate current American
medical policy trends as well as the policy directions not taken. What,
in short, are the straightforward implications for medical care of the
argument about welfare state developments introduced at the outset of
this chapter?

That argument, simply put, is that the broader politics of America's
reaction to stagflation (and later the budget deficit) have dominated
American health politics in the past two decades and more. For those
who concentrate on disputes within the medical polity, attention has
centered on the regulatory disappointments of the 1970s, the emergence
of cost containment as a preoccupation (even obsession), and the much-
noted disputes over the relative merits of regulatory versus so-called
competitive strategies in reforming an expensive, troubled American
medical world. These phenomena, undeniable at the surface of discussion, constitute for these purposes the consequences as much as the
causes of American health developments.

Macroeconomic events—the inflation of the Vietnam years and the
stagflation that worsened after the 1973–1974 oil crisis—set the direction
of social policy response but did not determine the particular shape.
The economy required restraint; that restraint was achieved differently
and to varying degrees in the welfare state economies of the OECD. The
American political response to the economic strains was one of a widespread sense of crisis in social policy, the overreaction to which Klein
and O'Higgins refer. The definition of the problem as one of crisis meant
that as the low growth of the economy reduced revenues and the tax cuts
of 1981 coupled with the arms buildup of the Carter-Reagan years
produced large deficits, new initiatives like national health insurance
became increasingly unthinkable at that time. Deficits, a large defense
budget, and the political unwillingness to raise taxes put medical care
policy in a paralytic vise. Only policy proposals that promised reductions in federal expenditure—like the heralded DRG innovation in Medicare hospital reimbursement (1983)—were on the agenda of active discussion. Otherwise social policy energy concentrated on protecting
current programs from further budget cutbacks. And the Gramm-Rud-

man-Hollings Act of 1985 institutionalized the politics of constraint, making large-scale programmatic innovation practically impossible.

The crisis formulation of the 1970s put medical care reformers on the defensive; the deficit politics of the 1980s boxed discussion still more tightly. The United States is, by international comparison, well known as a big spender for medical care. The 14 percent of GNP that is now expended for medical care results from widespread third-party payments, public and private. This fragmented and expensive system leaves sizable proportions of the society under- or uninsured. Access problems are bound to worsen as state health programs, federal programs, and private employers compete to shift costs to other parties, driving as hard a bargain as they can with beleaguered providers and insurers. Within the federal Medicare program, the debate hovers between those intent on increasing the out-of-pocket expenses and those who favor stricter limits on what medical providers can charge. It is rare to find serious discussion of recasting the program as a whole so as to extract a better bargain for the $70 billion level of expenditures.

I have characterized the welfare state debate in the United States as the triumph of rhetoric over reality. For the world of medical care, that triumph was evident in two of the most common disputes of the past decade or two: regulation versus competition and the related cost-control debate. In both instances, the broader reaction to the welfare state's troubles conditioned the struggle within medicine.

The competition/regulation dichotomy makes little analytical sense. There is no form of competition that does not rest on rules that enforce price competition as the central way in which suppliers gain customers. Equally, there is no form of state regulation that obliterates competition among providers for customers, prestige, favor, and honor. The dispute over competition and regulation is in fact over what form of competitive regulation is desirable and what its consequences will be for equity of access, fairness of finance, and quality of care. In developing this rhetorical dichotomy, American political discourse set itself apart from the rest of the OECD world. But that divergence in turn resulted from the peculiar American interpretation of the welfare state strains of the stagflation era as a crisis requiring retrenchment and precluding creative or flexible use of resources to meet changing needs.

The American form of cost-control disputes is equally distinctive. It is widely believed that governmental insurance triggered medical care inflation in the 1960s and that only the rigors of competition will restrain this failing industry. Again the broader context of cross-national findings makes one skeptical of the claim. In the rest of the OECD world, medical expenditures were the subject of considerable tinkering and restraint, but nowhere was there a major transformation of the postwar models of universal health coverage under public auspices. In these nations, increased expenditures in public medical programs were and are of great concern. But since the public programs are near-monopsonistic purchasers of care, the decision to reduce services affects all citizens directly. In the American case, the central state is but one payer (or purchaser). It has become a participant in the scramble to spread the inflated costs of medical care to other budgets. In Medicare, for example, the cost-control effort is directed at reducing federal deficits, permitting costs to spill onto other actors, whether they are the elderly, the providers, or other payers.

The turbulent world of medical care in the 1980s was, in my view, not the product of forces internal to medicine. Having come late to the welfare state's expansion, and having done so in the context of economic abundance and ideological hesitancy, the American polity was exceedingly ill prepared for the strains of the 1970s. In the 1980s we lived with the debris.

Chapter 4
Nonprofit Organizations and Health Care

WITH MARK SCHLESINGER AND
RICHARD W. SMITHEY

The topic of this chapter—nonprofits and medical care—is mired in controversy. Comparisons of the historical roles of nonprofit, governmental, and for-profit health institutions have been contentious. And the appraisal of contemporary arrangements is marked by fundamental differences of value, perspective, and fact.

The history of nonprofits in American medicine has been variously portrayed. The nonprofit form for hospitals is undoubtedly the dominant legal organization today. Some interpret this as triumph over the profit-making small hospital. For others, however, the story describes an endangered species reeling under the competition of large hospital chains. Or they discern a changing balance among the different forms of hospitals and see convergence, not divergence, as the dominant

Reprinted by permission from Walter W. Powell, ed., *The Nonprofit Sector: A Research Handbook* (New Haven: Yale University Press, 1987), pp. 221–39. Copyright © 1987 by Yale University Press. An earlier version appeared in the *Yale Journal of Regulation*, Vol. 3 (Spring 1986), pp. 313–49.

We thank Rachel Wagner and Jonathan Sherman for their research assistance and helpful comments. Elizabeth Auld and Heleri Ziou attended to the problems of producing a finished manuscript with their usual skill and unusual dedication, for which the authors are grateful. Woody Powell offered many helpful editorial suggestions.

theme. As with hospitals, so with physicians. They are alternately regarded as profit-making entrepreneurs cloaked in the misleading rhetoric of service professionalism or as technically expert professionals resisting the commercial blandishments of corporate medicine (Relman 1980, 967–68; Yordy 1986, 32). These conflicting perspectives shape the character, tone, and policy conclusions of much of the scholarship about the history of American medicine (Gray 1985; Starr 1982; Evans 1984).

Historical controversy spills over into disputes about what is currently taking place in American medicine (Fox 1986). Change is everywhere reported (Goldsmith 1984; Gray 1983, 1985), but its dimensions, consequences, and meaning are bewildering. The supply of physicians is growing—a glut for some, a boon to competition for others. A new payment arrangement for hospitals, diagnosis-related groups (DRGs), introduces case reimbursement into Medicare for the whole nation and sets in motion thousands of specialists offering to assist hospitals—of all forms—in playing the new game. Within the for-profit hospital sector, the number of hospitals organized in chains doubled between 1973 and 1982, and large for-profit corporations now own and manage hospitals that used to be publicly run, controlled by nonprofit boards, or owned by physicians (Gray 1985, 10–12). Some nonprofit hospitals form themselves into large systems and imitate the new corporate manner (Gray 1985, 13).[1]

The merging of substantial health-related institutions is not restricted to hospitals. Symptomatic of the vertical integration taking place in the health field was the proposed 1985 merger of the for-profit Hospital Corporation of America (HCA) with American Hospital Supply (AHS), a multibillion-dollar fusion of health giants (largest in their respective sectors) that dominated the nation's newspaper front pages for a few days in March 1985.[2] And, to complicate matters, nonprofit hospitals themselves have increasingly taken to the corporate marketplace, spawning for-profit subsidiaries, seeking debt financing that differs from stocks and bonds in legal name only, and searching for ways to imitate insurance companies, consulting firms, and industrial park entrepreneurs (Gray 1985, 17–19).[3] Health maintenance organizations (HMOs), home health agencies, dialysis and urgent-care centers, and other extra-hospital forms are increasingly managed by large proprietary conglomerates. All this takes place in full view of the national media, which are delighted to repeat the passionate exchanges of defenders of various faiths: markets, governments, and voluntarism.[4] No wonder, then, that rational appraisal of where we are and where we are going is difficult.

That appraisal is as controversial as the history and contemporary portraiture. The nonprofit form is lauded or derided, seen as inherently inefficient or as a benevolent community institution, regarded as threatened or on the verge of recovery (Clark 1980; Clarkson 1972). The growth of for-profit chains prompts journalistic categorization, and the monikers produce an acronymic frenzy: AMI, PPO, HCA, DRG, VHA.[5] Arnold Relman's "New Medical Industrial Complex" (NMIC), modeled on President Eisenhower's dread military-industrial complex of the 1950s (Relman 1980, 963), is but the most inflammatory example. In a $400 billion industry, there is more than enough money to finance companies of public relations specialists and lobbyists, all of whom can be relied on to produce dear and dread emblems of a benevolent or beastly past, a wondrous or dangerous present, and a fearful or hopeful future.[6]

Do the nonprofits behave inefficiently, or do they provide useful services that the cream-skimming, profit-making competitors shun? Are doctors compromised by working in hospitals controlled by corporations seeking profit? Or is this debate mostly a battle over how to rationalize an industry that grew fat, sloppy, and uncontrollable in an era of increased subsidies for medical care, medical research, and medical tinkering? No study—of a hospital closing or a new technology in action—and few summaries of these issues manage to emerge without being cast in the language of good and evil, delight and doom, prudence and waste.

Change is apparent in contemporary medicine, and public policy must, if this change is to be humanely managed, adapt. But the character of the debate about the nonprofit form—and its competitors—has been sufficiently confused and ill considered that much of the controversy should be reconsidered. The debate has been both ideological—commercialism and profit versus service and professionalism—and practical—which form is more efficient? The challenge of public policy is to adapt public rules to the central realities of American medicine, not the shibboleths of shrill discourse. In the case of medicine, other things besides the form of legal ownership are more important in fashioning appropriate responses. And so, in a paradoxical way, the central conclusion of a chapter on nonprofits in medicine is that the environment facing decision makers in medical institutions and the rules by which they operate are more significant than what institutions call themselves on their legal charters.

This chapter aims to provide a more accurate and better balanced assessment of the role of nonprofit organizations in health. It addresses first the history of the nonprofit form in American medicine and attempts to set that story in the broader history of American medical care. It then sketches the current state of nonprofit health institutions. The next part addresses the role of nonprofits in an industry with a mix of nonprofits, for-profits, and government institutions, in light of some of the expected differences among these forms. It examines in detail arguments about the merits and disadvantages of the nonprofit and for-profit forms, emphasizing the paradigmatic claims about cost, quality, and access among the opposing camps and important writers. And finally, we present a concluding discussion.

THE NONPROFIT FORM IN AMERICAN MEDICINE

The ongoing debate over the proper ownership of health institutions has been complicated by an unfortunate tendency to equate profit making with market-based allocations of services, to equate the proprietary form with profit making, and to cast ownership-related issues as crucial to the future evolution of American medicine. This is partly attributable to our public policies, since a large portion of American health legislation has encouraged private nonprofit providers as an alternative to proprietary institutions. There may be strong reasons to favor more or less use of markets in allocating some health services. But these can be separated in principle and practice from analyses of the appropriate role of for-profit or nonprofit health care (Enthoven 1980; Dunham, Morone, & White 1982). Changes in the ownership mix of health care providers may well have some important implications for health policy, but completely eliminating either for-profit or nonprofit providers would in itself remedy few if any of the problems facing American medicine.

Casting the argument in terms of a choice between legal forms in medical care obscures the historical sources of the present situation. What we are witnessing is a heightening of an old and fundamental tension within medicine over whose interests should predominate. The steady pressure of rising costs, accompanied by the opportunities to earn high returns in medical care, has caused this tension to resurface. To understand the present, one must first comprehend the special features of medical care as an industry.

First, the relationship between provider and consumer of medical services differs, in several important ways, from that for other services. The asymmetry of information between the provider and the patient is more pronounced than for most services,[7] even in other areas in which nonprofit ownership is common. The importance of these asymmetries is heightened by the emotional associations of lifesaving treatment and the traumas of injury and dread disease. For many, it is crucial that the relationship between provider and patient be one of "care giving," for in no "business" except prostitution is the pursuit of profit alone seen as so antithetical to the professional relationship clients seek (Titmuss 1971).

These considerations have in part shaped the policies that constrain the practices of health professionals. The medical professions have gained unusual authority in the belief that professional norms and sanctions would appropriately limit medical behavior (Arrow 1963; Fox 1986). There have been extensive attempts to encourage the ethic of care giving—through education, honorific example, and nonmonetary rewards.[8]

The judgment that professional norms are insufficient to regulate the medical industry has led to extensive medical legislation (Starr 1982, 402; Brown 1986, 22–23). Some policies promote access to care by those disadvantaged in a private market. Others aim to control the cost and quality of the services that all patients receive (Ruchlin 1979; Drake 1980; Raffel 1980, 601–02). Many of these policies have been explicitly designed to promote nonprofit organizations, either by enforcing less stringent regulations on them or by providing subsidies not available to their for-profit counterparts. "Numerous statutes, regulations, and judicial doctrines," we are reminded, "discriminate against for-profit hospitals," including preferential access to construction grants, subsidies for training programs, and planning and operational assistance for a range of health services (Clark 1980, 1473).

Second, understanding the role of nonprofit organizations in health is also made more difficult by the complexity of medicine and the diversity of institutions providing services. Nonprofit organizations treat acute illness (for example, hospitals, health maintenance organizations, neighborhood health centers), palliate chronic conditions (home health agencies, nursing homes, renal dialysis centers), as well as provide supportive services such as insurance (Blue Cross, Blue Shield), education and lobbying (American Medical Association, American Hospital Association), and research (March of Dimes, American Cancer Society). The institutional missions and the roles of professionals vary greatly across these services. It would, therefore, not be surprising to find that the implications of ownership vary as well.

Medical care accounted for 60 percent of total charitable nonprofit organization revenues or expenditures in 1980 (Salamon & Abramson 1982, 15). And private nonprofit agencies, by the measure of dollar expenditure, dominate the provision of medical care. Such aggregated

Table 4.1
Relative proportions of for-profit, private nonprofit, and public health care providers in the United States, 1980

Institutions offering services	Measured in terms of—	Percentage of services provided by—		
		For-profit	Nonprofit	Public
Acute hospitals	Beds	8.5	69.6	21.9
Psychiatric hospitals	Beds	6.0	4.7	89.3
Nursing homes	Beds	67.6	21.3	11.0
Homes for mentally handicapped	Residents	46.2	37.7	16.5
Blood banks	Facilities	63.3	5.8	30.9
Dialysis centers	Facilities	38.5	44.3	17.2
Health maintenance organizations	Enrollees	15.8	84.2	NA
Health insurance	Enrollees	45.2	42.7	12.0
Home health agencies	Patients	25.5	64.1	10.4

Source: Schlesinger 1984.

pictures, however, mask considerable variation. The proportion of nonprofits differs greatly from one service to the next, as Table 4.1 illustrates. For some services, nonprofit institutions serve as much as three-quarters of all consumers, for others, less than 10 percent.

Nonprofit organizations may be classified by the way in which they are financed: donative (largely by philanthropy), or commercial (payments by clients and third-party insurers). Over the last century the trend in health has been for donative nonprofits to become commercial nonprofits (hospitals) and for support that had been donative to be increasingly assumed by government (medical research and education).[9] The histories and identities of these organizations have been shaped by changes in their financing—who paid them, how much, and by what methods. Other factors, such as demographic patterns and historical changes, have, of course, also influenced the location and character of nonprofits in the health industry.

The relative importance of nonprofit and for-profit health institutions has fluctuated over time. Services that are now dominated by nonprofit institutions, such as acute-care hospitals, were at one time predominantly investor owned. Services that now have a substantial proprietary sector, such as HMOs and renal dialysis facilities, only 20 or so years ago were almost exclusively provided by private nonprofit and public agencies (Schlesinger 1984, 80). These historical fluctuations suggest that diverse and interrelated factors determine the scale and role of nonprofit enterprise in medical care. Three distinct historical periods of change in mix and ownership form throughout the medical care industry emerge from our investigations.

1900–1950: The Institutionalization of Health Care and the Dominance of Nonprofit Organizations

Throughout most of the nineteenth century, medical care was largely a cottage industry. Hospitals were principally facilities for caring for the sickly poor; those with higher incomes were treated at home by physicians. Hospitals and physicians coexisted, the former supported by religious organizations and government subsidies, the latter by fees from patients (Raffel 1980, 241–46; Starr 1982, 145–79; Stevens 1982, 552–55). Because of their religious affiliations, most of the hospitals established during this period were nonprofit. Toward the end of the nineteenth century, however, the practice of medicine became more complex. Medical education was increasingly specialized and a number of new medical schools were opened. Hospitals evolved into the primary setting for treating the very ill and began to require patient fees for support (Starr 1982, 157–61).

In this evolution, for-profit and nonprofit hospitals retained many of the distinctions that had previously existed between doctors and hospitals. The for-profit facilities continued for the most part to be operated by a single doctor or small group of physicians and to cater to wealthier patients (Starr 1982, 165). The usually larger nonprofit hospitals continued to rely heavily on philanthropic support. The absence or presence of philanthropy led to pronounced regional variations in ownership mix. The East and Midwest, populated by service-oriented religious groups and philanthropically minded capitalists, were dominated by nonprofit hospitals. The West, however, lacked a strong philanthropic tradition, having been settled after hospitals had begun to rely more heavily on patient fees for support and after the charitable mission of care for the poor was no longer the hospital's central function. Here, for-profit hospitals were far more common (Starr 1982, 170–71).

During the late nineteenth century a rapid proliferation of proprietary hospitals and medical schools took place as the country grew to the west (Stevens 1971, 24–25). The growth of nonprofit facilities was further inhibited because state and local governments withdrew subsidies that had previously been available (Stevens 1982, 560). By 1900, this growth of proprietary institutions had significantly changed the ownership picture in American medicine: over half of the medical schools and 60 percent of the hospitals in operation were privately owned, in most cases by one doctor (Bays 1983b). There was not yet a technological justification for large hospitals and usually the small proprietary hospital/clinic corresponded well to the then-dominant solo practice (Bays 1983b).

The subsequent fifty years brought increased formalization, standardization, and institutionalization to American medicine. During the first several decades of this century, this pattern was reflected primarily in the emergence of a standardized, more technically oriented set of medical schools, hospitals, and to a lesser extent, nursing homes. The increasing complexity of medical care raised the cost of both medical training and treatment, creating a greater need for subsidization (Starr 1982, 118). This in turn favored the growth of new nonprofit institutions that could tap religious affiliations (Starr 1982, 169ff.; Vladeck 1980), offer tax deductions in return for donations, and remain largely exempted from growing government regulation (Nielsen 1979, 184).

A large proportion of the medical profession strongly favored the nonprofit form. The increased emphasis on technical aspects of medicine and the institutions' dependence on fee-paying patients allowed doctors to increase their authority to the point where they became the dominant decision makers in hospitals (Starr 1982, 161). Rejecting for-profit enterprise reduced the threat of corporate control on this authority (Starr 1982, 218). Since antitrust laws were only loosely applied, nonprofit institutions also provided a way to control entry into medicine and to enhance the financial returns of a medical practice (Horty & Mulholland 1983; Weller 1984, 1351–92).

The combined influence of economic incentives and professional interest thus led to a diminished role for proprietary institutions. By the mid-1920s, proprietary medical schools were starting to disappear, the proportion of investor-owned hospitals had declined to just over a third, and virtually all the medically oriented nursing homes were nonprofit (Bays 1983b, 367; Vladeck 1980).[10] The remaining for-profit institutions were disproportionately located in rapidly growing areas, where population increased faster than philanthropic voluntarism could supply new capital (Steinwald & Neuhauser 1970, 819–20) or where the philanthropic tradition was weak.

This trend was reinforced, in the short run, by the introduction of health insurance during the early 1930s (Raffel 1980, 393–94; Starr 1982, 295–98). Faced with financially strained hospitals and proposals for national health insurance, the American Medical Association abandoned its earlier rigid opposition to hospital insurance (Nielsen 1979, 112). With the cooperation of the American Hospital Association and enabling legislation passed by state governments (Rorem 1939; Law 1974, 8–11), Blue Cross and later Blue Shield were established to offer hospital and medical insurance, respectively.

Both of these provider-sponsored plans were organized as nonprofit enterprises for several reasons. Physician autonomy was, as noted before, less threatened by the nonprofit corporate form.[11] In addition, the insurance plans worked closely with providers. Proprietary ownership of these health insurance companies might well have raised questions about the appropriateness of the nonprofit status of hospitals.[12] Finally, state enabling legislation granted to the Blues what were effectively state-sanctioned monopolies in providing service-benefit plans (Law 1974, 8ff.). Legislators no doubt favored nonprofit ownership in part to avoid the appearance of having sanctioned organizations that could extract near-monopoly "profits" from the health industry (Law 1974, 11).

The appropriate legal status of these health insurance plans was a matter of considerable dispute. Half the states refused to grant the plans tax-exempt status, and the Internal Revenue Service ruled that donations to the plans were not tax deductible.[13] To bolster their claim to nonprofit status, the Blues adopted the policy of community rating— charging all residents of a community the same premium. This effectively subsidized the old and the poor, who had higher than average medical expenses—at least those who could afford to purchase insurance.[14]

The growth of Blue Cross and Blue Shield reinforced the dominant position of nonprofit organizations in medicine. By the early 1940s, nonprofit plans controlled more than two-thirds of the health insurance market (Schlesinger 1984, 79). Blue Cross negotiated lower reimbursement rates for proprietary hospitals than for their nonprofit counterparts. This accelerated the decline of investor-owned facilities: by 1946 they represented less than 10 percent of all hospitals (Steinwald & Neuhauser 1970, 819). In addition, nonprofit hospitals, faced with the loss of more lucrative patients to proprietary hospitals, relaxed their previous strict staff admission policies and absorbed physicians from proprietary hospitals (Starr 1982, 165–71). Physicians remained uncontested in their authority to control both the delivery and the financing of medical care, authority mediated first by the nonprofit hospitals and later by Blue Cross and Blue Shield. Nevertheless, the growth of insurance under the auspices of the Blues was to sow the seeds of the eventual rebirth of proprietary institutions in medicine.

1950–1975: Public Subsidies and the Renaissance of Proprietary Health Care

Following World War II, some federal policymakers became increasingly concerned with encouraging access to medical care. To this end, legislation was passed subsidizing the medical industry (Lave & Lave 1974; Rosenblatt 1978, 264–70). At first, funds were paid directly to providers who agreed to care for the poor. Later subsidies were directed at increasing the effective demand of patients for medical care: unsuccessful attempts at national health insurance in the 1940s precipitated the drive in the 1950s for government health insurance covering the elderly—the Medicare program eventually enacted in 1965 (Marmor 1973, 13–16).

Initially, the direct public financing of facilities tended to enhance the position of nonprofit institutions. In fact, many financing programs were specifically designed to do so, by making funds available either exclusively or preferentially to private nonprofit or public agencies. The postwar Hill-Burton program, for example, subsidized construction of a variety of nonprofit and public health care facilities, though funds were allocated primarily to the construction of short-term general hospitals. Hill-Burton subsidized one-third of all hospital construction projects between 1947 and 1972, supplying about 10 percent of the total capital costs (Lave & Lave 1974, 16).

Because nonprofit agencies were relatively slow to respond to subsidies, however, their share of services increased only marginally as a result of these funds (Vladeck 1980, 41–42; Lave & Lave 1974, 45). Moreover, by stimulating the expansion of public facilities, government subsidies indirectly altered and to some extent undermined the traditional role of private nonprofit medical care. Health institutions operated by state and local government grew rapidly during this period. Between 1945 and 1960, beds in short-term public hospitals increased by 15 percent, in psychiatric hospitals by 20 percent, and in nursing homes by over 200 percent.[15]

Table 4.2
Public subsidies and the growth of for-profit health care

Type of facility	Change in coverage	Market share of proprietary agencies (percent)	
		3–5 years before	3–5 years after
Acute hospitals	Medicare enacted 1965	5	7
Nursing homes	Medicaid enacted 1965	60	70
Dialysis centers	Medicare covered 1972	4	21
Home health agencies	Medicare covered 1981	7	25
Psychiatric hospitals	Private insurance coverage mandated by states 1975–80	1	6
Residences for mentally impaired	Title XX enacted 1974	10	38

Source: Schlesinger 1984.

The growth of public medical facilities shifted much of the responsibility for caring for the poor to these institutions and away from their private nonprofit counterparts (Gage 1985, 77; Feder, Hadley, & Mullner 1984). This shift, coupled with the availability of public funds for capital projects, reduced the apparent need for donative financing, itself one of the chief justifications for nonprofit status.

In the 1960s and continuing through the mid-1970s, governmental program subsidies expanded from facilities to health insurance and direct payment for care. The passage of Medicare and Medicaid in 1965 (Marmor 1973; Stevens & Stevens 1974) and amendments to Social Security in 1972 and 1974 reflected this development and had a significant impact on the mix of ownership in American medicine (see Table 4.2).

Rapidly growing health insurance—public and private—has almost invariably led to an increased proportion of services provided by proprietary institutions (Vladeck 1980, 105). The reasons for this are complex, but they probably reflect both organizational conflicts within nonprofit agencies and the ability of investor-owned organizations to acquire capital more rapidly (Steinwald & Neuhauser 1970, 828). What-ever the causes, the link between increasing health insurance coverage and an expanded role for proprietary organizations is striking.

This pattern was first evident in the health insurance industry itself. Wage freezes during World War II and the Korean War prompted unions to push for increases in nonwage benefits. The most prominent growth took place in health insurance, with the number of enrollees growing sharply from less than 13 million in 1940 to over 100 million in 1955 (Schlesinger 1984, 79). With this growth in health insurance coverage, the market share of commercial insurers increased from 37 percent in 1940 to 55 percent in 1960.

The growth of proprietary providers was even more pronounced after the enactment in 1965 of Medicare and Medicaid (Table 4.2). Initial implementation of these two programs boosted the amount of services (relative to nonprofits) provided by investor-owned hospitals and nurs-ing homes, respectively (Starr 1982, 434). The subsequent expansion of Medicare benefits in the 1970s encouraged the growth of for-profit renal dialysis centers and home health agencies, and similar expansions of investor-owned psychiatric facilities resulted from other public financ-ing.[16]

The expansion of investor-owned insurers increased competitive pressures on nonprofit insurance organizations. Commercial insurers offered policies based on the experience of particular groups rather than the overall health care use in the community. For groups with below-average risk of illness, including many employee groups, this experience rating offered much lower premiums than did community rating. During the 1950s a number of employee groups shifted from the Blues to commercial carriers, and others threatened to do so. In the face of this competitive pressure, the Blues virtually abandoned community rating by the 1960s, eliminating the implicit subsidy to high-risk individuals (Krizay & Wilson 1974, 40).

This was but the first example of a number of changes in the services offered by nonprofit health providers when faced with competition from investor-owned institutions. The breadth and significance of these changes, however, became apparent only in combination with additional changes in American medicine that occurred in subsequent years.

The impact of Medicare and Medicaid was far more profound than simply stimulating the resurgence of for-profit enterprises in American medicine. Together with the growth of private health insurance, Medi-care and Medicaid sharply increased the flow of funds into the health industry. Third-party financing, in short, transformed medicine into a virtual gold mine for commercial nonprofit as well as for-profit enterprises.

The relative position of Blue Cross also improved as a result of Medicare. The implicit designation of Blue Cross as the dominant fiscal intermediary for Medicare's hospital plan had eased the bill's passage in 1965; this concession signified an accommodating disposition toward hospitals and physicians in Medicare's first years of operation (Starr 1982, 375; Feder 1977, 37; Marmor 1973, 141). Moreover, Blue Cross's cost-based scheme of hospital reimbursement, transferred nearly intact to Medicare, meant that Blue Cross assumed a far more important position than when it was simply in the business of selling group hospitalization insurance (Law 1974, 93–102).

Third-party payment was a key transformative factor for American medicine. Blue Cross and Blue Shield, like hospitals, did little to threaten the autonomy of physicians. The benign nature of Medicare's early administration and the regularity of its payment reinforced the earlier patterns of third-party private insurers. The result was that, both before and after Medicare's passage, the authoritative power to determine medical costs still lay within the medical profession, whose interests continued to be furthered through Blue Cross, although in less direct ways.

Government health insurance prompted a period of extended growth for American medical institutions. Medicare permitted generous depreciation allowances for capital and, by reimbursing capital costs which were then plowed back into the cost base, inserted an inflationary factor into its own payments, which were then determined by the provider-dominated insurers (Feder 1977, 113–17). It was thus no surprise that the rate of medical inflation rose to twice the annual increases in the consumer price index for the period 1966–1972 (Marmor, Wittman, & Heagy 1983).

High levels of medical inflation continued through the 1970s (see Table 4.3) as efforts for reform concentrated on new forms of health regulation and new methods of delivering care. Regulatory initiatives, Professional Standards Review Organizations (PSROs) and Health Systems Agencies (HSAs) among them, were begun with national health insurance in mind. National health insurance, however, never materialized, and both the federal government and the health industry were left with a fragmented set of controls. The inflationary forces at work in medicine—principally broad health insurance coverage, pluralistic financing, and weak countervailing regulatory authorities—worked their

Table 4.3
National health expenditures

Calendar year	Total amount (billions)	Percentage of GNP[a]
1960	$26.9	5.3
1970	74.7	7.5
1980	249.0	9.5
1981	286.6	9.8
1982	322.4	10.5
1983	355.4	10.8

Source: Freeland and Schendler 1984.
a. GNP = Gross National Product.

will through the 1970s (Brown 1985). The decade began with marked medical inflation, witnessed frustrated public reform, and ended with a strong mandate for cost control in Washington (Starr & Marmor 1984).[17]

Confident as the center of scientific progress, financially rewarded, and imbued with considerable cultural authority, American medicine had experienced a golden age in the quarter century after World War II. But events of the period since 1965 have changed the industry's outlook. Inflationary concerns grew to a crescendo in the late 1970s, and several initiatives designed to bring access, cost, and humane health care into a reasonable equilibrium were almost all disappointing. It was in the context of the mid-1970s that the debate over the role and character of the nonprofit institution in health sharply increased.

1975–1985: The Era of Cost Containment and Increased Competition

Policymakers' and Americans' increasing concern about medical inflation led to direct changes in the health industry—the growth of the prospective-payment system, the increased consolidation of insurance and service delivery within prepaid health plans, and the imposition of a variety of regulatory measures. Inflation also had some indirect effects. These included threats to the financial stability of government-operated health facilities and subtle shifts in popular expectations about the responsibility of health facilities to their local communities. Most pervasive, and perhaps most important as an influence on the roles of nonprofit and for-profit health providers, was the increased price competition among suppliers of medical services.

This competition took a number of forms. A variety of negotiated arrangements, including "preferred provider" and "exclusive provider" agreements, were established to channel patients to a single or small group of providers, in return for price discounts (Gabel & Ermann 1985). More active negotiation by third-party payers over prices eroded the ability of hospitals to cross-subsidize particular types of care and patients (Sloan & Becker 1984, 677–78; Clark 1980, 1480–81). Health maintenance organizations—which historically have had lower rates of hospitalization and costs—grew substantially, with enrollment increasing from less than 6 million in 1975 to over 12 million in 1983.[18]

These sectorwide increases in competition have had significant implications for the role of private nonprofit providers. On the one hand, diminished cross-subsidization of patients and services reduced the ability of nonprofit institutions to offer unprofitable services, which had previously distinguished them from their for-profit counterparts (Schlesinger & Dorwart 1984). On the other hand, the loss of cross-subsidization and increased dumping of the sickest patients from private facilities threatened the financial stability of many public institutions (Feder & Hadley 1985, 70). Between 1977 and 1983, 128 short-term hospitals operated by state and local governments were closed, a decline of 7 percent (American Hospital Association 1983). Ironically, the need for a charitable role for private health institutions seemed to be growing at exactly the time when nonprofit organizations were least willing to meet that need.

At the same time, there has been a subtle shift in popular expectations about the responsibilities of health providers. Patients in the past have placed considerable trust in a physician's competence and expected fiduciary responsibility from physicians. This trust seems to be eroding as the service ethic in health care has become demythologized and a more commercially oriented ethic has developed among providers. These changes have been accompanied by a loss of professional authority and autonomy; some of the power once wielded by physicians has shifted to those who previously supported them—the financial and operating officers of hospitals, prepaid group practices, and both Blue Cross and Blue Shield.

Increased competition and lessened professional autonomy have reduced or eliminated some of the goals and practices that once distinguished nonprofit and for-profit providers of health care. Nonprofit institutions increasingly mirror the institutional structure of their investor-owned competitors; they have established holding companies, for-profit subsidiaries, multifacility chains, and more overtly hierarchical organizations that create a stronger role and added discretion for non-physician managers. As with the Blues in the late 1950s, practices of nonprofit and for-profit health care facilities have converged in many ways. At the 1985 annual meetings of the American Psychiatric Association, for example, Leon Eisenberg of Harvard Medical School observed:

> The worst of it is that voluntaries, unable to cross-subsidize expensive but essential clinical services because of cost-competition, are becoming less distinguishable from the proprietaries, as they "market," and worse, "demarket," "diversify," "unbundle," "spin-off" for-profit subsidiaries, develop "convenience-oriented feeder systems," attempt to adjust case mix and triage admissions by their ability to pay.

Summary: Historical Perspectives on the Role of Nonprofit Health Care Providers

Our historical review suggests several important patterns in and influences on the role of nonprofits in the health world. For one thing, for each service there appears to be a life cycle in the role of nonprofit providers. As new services develop, through technological or social innovation, the initial pioneers are almost always private nonprofit agencies. This is in part because new services are typically expensive and require subsidization from public or philanthropic donations or other sources. Most likely, it reflects as well the importance of nonpecuniary goals for the most innovative providers.

As a health service gains broader acceptance, however, two important changes occur. First its use in the proprietary sector increases.[19] If the increase is sufficiently rapid, existing nonprofit providers may be unable to expand expeditiously to provide additional services. The resulting entry of proprietary institutions creates competitive pressures that tend to bring about a convergence between the behaviors of non-profit and for-profit providers. And, second, policymakers become concerned with ensuring adequate access for those unable to pay for the service. This concern leads them to provide subsidies to public agencies to finance the poor and uninsured, which in turn tends to reduce the importance of charitable provision of care by private nonprofit agencies.

To understand the role of nonprofit medical care providers, then, it is important to know where a particular service lies in this life cycle. For the health sector as a whole, there will be some services at early stages, some at intermediate, and some at later stages. For example, HMOs are moving from the first to the second stage, and hospitals are entering the later stages.

The implications of ownership for the performance of health institutions depend most significantly on professionals, particularly physicians. This is evident, most crudely, in the relationship between the extent of physician involvement in delivery of care and the extent to which for-profit organizations are active in a particular service. As shown in Table 4.1, for example, the services in which doctors play the least important role—health insurance, nursing homes, blood banks, and residences for the mentally impaired—are those in which proprietary enterprises deliver the largest portion of services.

There may thus be an important link between professional incentives and authority and the role of nonprofit health care facilities. The normative implications of this relationship have been the subject of much debate. Some view the physician's authority in nonprofit agencies as essentially elitist, reflecting goals that diverge from other important social values (Clark 1980, 1439). Others see this same interaction as a means of preserving important nonmonetary social ends, including access to care for the poor, avoidance of undesirable low-quality care, and the promotion of a stronger fiduciary relationship between health institutions and the communities in which they are located (Relman 1980, 967–68).

To better understand the extent and ways in which competition between nonprofits and for-profits has led to a convergence in their practices and to better grasp the interaction of professional incentives and ownership, it is useful to review the literature on the comparative performance of contemporary for-profit and nonprofit health care institutions.

COMPARATIVE STUDIES OF NONPROFIT AND FOR-PROFIT HEALTH INSTITUTIONS: THE EVIDENCE

American health policy has concentrated on three primary aims: limiting the cost of treatment, ensuring the provision of services of adequate quality, and promoting access to care. Past studies of the effects of ownership on the behavior of providers have understandably focused on these three areas.

Ownership and Medical Costs

Two substantial sets of empirical studies have been conducted on the relationship between ownership and economic performance—the first focusing on nursing homes, the second on short-term general hospitals. Over a dozen studies have compared average costs of care in nonprofit and for-profit nursing homes.[20] Using varying data bases and measures of costs, these studies have reached a common conclusion: controlling for characteristics of patients, range of services provided, and other attributes of the facility, for-profit homes have average costs 5 to 15 percent lower than their nonprofit counterparts.

In contrast, investigations of the hospital industry have found only small, inconsistent differences in reported costs of proprietary and nonprofit facilities. Cost per day is usually higher in for-profit facilities. But shorter lengths of stay have led to their relative cost per admission being measured as lower in some studies, higher in others, and roughly equal in the rest (Sloan & Becker 1984; Ermann & Gabel 1984; Pattison & Katz 1983; Sloan & Vraciu 1983, 34; Lewin, Derzon, & Margulies 1981, 52; Bays 1979).

This research also seems to indicate ownership-related differences in costs in facilities where physicians' roles are relatively attenuated (Koetting 1980), but not where there is a stronger professional presence.[21] This suggests that professional standards and incentives mitigate some of the incentives for cost reduction (either through increased efficiency or reduced quality) that might otherwise be associated with for-profit ownership.

Ownership and the Quality of Medical Care

Assessments of ownership-related differences in quality for the most part mirror the findings on cost of care. For those facilities in which physicians control the delivery of care, there seem to be few if any measurable differences in quality (Schlesinger & Dorwart 1984, 959; Schlesinger 1985, 11). For example, a recent review concluded that there is no evidence that the profit motive induces physicians to compromise quality: "Unless new definitions of quality are proposed which are more rigorous, comprehensible, measurable, and widely acceptable than those noted above, there appears to be no basis for examining this dimension beyond the results of existing studies" (Sherman & Chilingerian 1984, 5).

On the other hand, where physicians play a less active role, the evidence suggests that lower-quality care is found in for-profit settings. Whether there are differences in the *average* quality is a matter of debate.[22] There is fairly consistent evidence, however, that for-profit facilities are disproportionately represented among institutions offering the very lowest quality care (Vladeck 1980, 123; Smith 1981, 86; Koetting 1980, 18).

Ownership and Access to Medical Care

Throughout their history, for-profit institutions have labored under the suspicion that they treat only the more profitable patients. In 1970 it was noted that "the most serious indictment of proprietary hospitals is contained in the argument that has been labeled 'cream-skimming'" (Steinwald & Neuhauser 1970, 832).[23] Almost 25 years later, the scale of proprietary operations has enlarged greatly, but the concerns of observers have not changed. The quest for profits is regarded as "an additional motive to private provider groups and institutions to engage in patient skimming and to discontinue needed but cost-ineffective services" (Nutter 1984, 918).

Private nonprofit institutions, however, are also reported to select carefully the patients they treat. In the mid-1970s, the National Health and Environmental Law Project received a number of reports from local legal service programs indicating significant channeling of "indigent patients who present themselves for treatment at private nonprofit hospital emergency rooms to municipal and county hospitals" (Silver 1974, 184). Based on these and other reports, some analysts have concluded that cream skimming is a major factor within the voluntary sector as well: "The suburban community hospitals avoid the poor. . . . The voluntary teaching hospitals prefer if they can to take the 'interesting cases' and send everyone else to the city or county hospital" (Neuhauser 1974, 240).

It is clear then that private nonprofit and for-profit health providers each engage in some screening of patients who seek care. If ownership affects restrictions on access, it will thus be reflected not in the presence but in the nature or extent of patient selection. Facilities may select among patients to further a variety of organizational objectives, including increased surplus (profits) or enhanced status as teaching or research institutions. We focus here on selection of patients on the basis of profitability, since this can be most readily measured.

Providers of medical care can avoid unprofitable patients in three ways. First, facilities can simply be located away from low-income areas. Second, they can choose not to provide services used dispro-portionately by the uninsured or underinsured. Third, they can actively screen for and discourage admission by those unable to pay for care. This screening can be accomplished by requiring a means test prior to admission or by not offering sliding fee scales for patients unable to cover fully the costs of care. Evidence from past studies suggests that for-profit providers are more likely to use each of these methods, and that this occurs both for facilities in which physicians play an important role and for those in which they do not.

Screening and Location of the Facility To the extent that facilities avoid patients with limited ability to pay, one would expect them to locate in affluent areas. If for-profit providers are more sensitive to these incentives, they should provide a higher proportion of services in these areas than in less profitable localities. Most studies of the relationship between ownership and choice of location examine the location patterns of short-term general hospitals. These studies have in fact found that the share of services provided under proprietary auspices is highest in states with high per capita income (Kushman & Nuckton 1977, 201), rapidly increasing levels of income (Steinwald & Neuhauser 1970, 828), and extensive insurance coverage (Bays 1983a, 955). These patterns persist whether one focuses on all for-profit hospitals or just those associated with multifacility chains (Mullner & Hadley 1984, 149). Similar patterns are seen within states, with investor-owned facilities disproportionately located in counties that have relatively few Medicaid patients (Homer, Bradham, & Rushefsky 1984).

Less research has been done on other types of care. However, for-profit psychiatric inpatient care is three times higher in states where private coverage for this care is required, and for-profit home health care is almost three times more prevalent in states with generous Med-icaid programs (Schlesinger & Blumenthal 1986). (See Table 4.4.)

Screening and Selection of Services To screen out patients with limited ability to pay, a facility can be expected to avoid offering two types of services: (1) those that are not reimbursed or are under-reimbursed by insurance plans, and (2) those that are used dispropor-tionately by patients who are uninsured or covered by Medicaid (Sloan & Becker 1984).

Psychiatric hospitals provide several good examples of the first type of service. Emergency telephone and suicide prevention services are generally unreimbursed, since the client is often unidentified and there-

Table 4.4
Insurance coverage and market shares of proprietary health care facilities,
1980

	Proportion of facilities that are for-profit	
Type of facility	States that mandate psychiatric inpatient coverage in private insurance[a]	States with no mandate
Psychiatric hospitals	42.9%	13.4%
	States with generous Medicaid programs[b]	States with less generous Medicaid programs
Home health agencies	8.3%	3.3%
	States with special ESRD Medicaid coverage[c]	States with no Medicaid ESRD[d] program
Dialysis centers	30.7%	24.5%

Source: Schlesinger and Blumenthal 1986.
a. Twenty-two states.
b. Twenty-one states in which Medicaid fees for specialists equal at least 90 percent of Medicaid reimbursement.
c. Thirty-six states.
d. End-stage renal disease.

fore cannot be billed. Home care and day care programs tend, for historical reasons, to be underreimbursed by insurers (Schlesinger & Dorwart 1984, 963). Facilities that screen on ability to pay would therefore tend to avoid such services, and, indeed, surveys of psychiatric hospitals show that for-profit institutions are four to five times less likely to offer such services than are either their private nonprofit or public counterparts (Schlesinger & Dorwart 1984, 964). A study of outpatient services in general hospitals found that for-profit facilities, particularly those affiliated with a multihospital corporation, were less likely to offer unprofitable services (Shortell et al. 1986).

Facilities that select patients on ability to pay can also be expected to avoid those services that are used disproportionately by the indigent. Low-income patients are apt to be either uninsured or covered by Medicaid, which in most states pays hospitals at a rate far lower than reimbursement from other insurers (Sloan & Becker 1984, 682).[24] In

Table 4.5
Percentages of hospitals with low-income services available, in urban areas
with both private nonprofit and for-profit short-term general hospitals, 1980

	Type of service				
				Chemical dependency unit	
Type of hospital	Psychiatric outpatient	Outpatient department	Dental	Inpatient	Outpatient
100–199 beds					
For-profit	6.3	35.4	31.3	12.5	10.4
Private, nonprofit	8.9	57.1	44.4	26.7	26.7
200–299 beds					
For-profit	16.7	41.7	41.7	4.2	4.2
Private, nonprofit	19.12	60.0	48.9	14.9	14.9

Source: Schlesinger and Blumenthal 1986.
Note: Statistics are based on hospitals in Anaheim, Atlanta, Augusta,
Chattanooga, Chicago, Corpus Christi, Dallas, El Paso, Fort Worth, Houston,
Little Rock, Los Angeles, Louisville, Memphis, Miami, Mobile, Montgomery,
Nashville, New Orleans, New York, Phoenix, Richmond, Saint Petersburg,
San Antonio, San Diego, San Francisco, Seattle, and Tucson.

short-term general hospitals—where data on service mix are most readily available—investor-owned hospitals are again significantly less likely
to offer such services (Schlesinger & Blumenthal 1986). Controlling for
size and local characteristics, private nonprofit hospitals are significantly more likely to adopt services used by indigent patients (Cromwell
& Kanak 1982; Schlesinger & Blumenthal 1986). (See Table 4.5.) Where
a hospital is the sole local institution, these differences in behavior are
smaller (Schlesinger & Blumenthal 1986, 12).

     Screening and Admissions Policies Admissions policies can
influence the average ability to pay in a facility in two ways. First,
exclusionary policies (for example, requiring a means test) can be used
to screen out particular classes of payers, such as the uninsured or
those covered by Medicaid. Second, by providing services at a reduced
charge, facilities can encourage the patronage of lower-income patients.
Facilities that seek more profitable patients can be expected to adopt
the former policies but avoid the latter.
    For-profit institutions appear significantly more likely to fit this pat-

Table 4.6
Proportion of physicians reporting exclusions of patients of various types,
1980

Independent physicians:

Type of patient	Public	Nonprofit	For-profit
Uninsured	0.14	0.20	0.43
Medicaid	0.03	0.05	0.15
Medicare	0.02	0.01	0.04

System-affiliated physicians:

Type of patient	Public	Nonprofit	For-profit
Uninsured	0.09	0.19	0.52
Medicaid	0.03	0.05	0.16
Medicare	0.01	0.01	0.05

Source: Schlesinger and Blumenthal 1986.

tern. Surveys of physicians reveal that investor-owned hospitals are two to three times as likely to adopt policies to discourage admissions of uninsured or Medicaid patients (Schlesinger & Blumenthal 1986, 14). (See Table 4.6.) Conversely, a survey of long-term care facilities, including nursing homes, psychiatric hospitals, and institutions for the mentally handicapped, found that proprietary facilities were one-half to one-quarter as likely to offer services at reduced charge as were their nonprofit counterparts (Schlesinger & Blumenthal 1986).[25] (See Table 4.7.)

Discussion of the Empirical Findings

These findings suggest that ownership does influence facility performance. Differences in cost and quality of care were confined largely to institutions in which physicians play a minor role. However, virtually all investor-owned institutions appear more likely to select patients on the basis of their ability to pay. For-profit facilities are also more likely to locate in areas with higher incomes and to avoid offering services used most by indigent patients. And proprietary providers appear more likely to screen patients on insurance status and less likely

Table 4.7
Level of charges as a reason for selection of long-term care facilities, 1980

	Ownership of facility		
	Proprietary	Nonprofit	Public

A. Percentage of administrators responding that the availability of service at no charge was an important reason for the selection of their facility by consumers.

	Proprietary	Nonprofit	Public
Psychiatric hospitals	11.2	27.3	34.9
Institutions for mentally handicapped	15.5	22.2	48.2
Nursing homes	6.6	22.2	48.7

B. Percentage of clients responding that the availability of service at reduced or no charge was an important reason for their selection of a facility.

	Proprietary	Nonprofit	Public
Psychiatric hospitals	4.7	9.0	16.7
Institution for mentally handicapped	8.0	12.6	20.7
Nursing homes	4.9	8.9	23.8

Source: Schlesinger 1985.

to encourage patronage by low-income patients by offering sliding fee scales.

The evidence concerning selection on the basis of cost of care is considerably weaker, in part because there are relatively few data on access under prospective reimbursement. The evidence that does exist is consistent with the conclusion that proprietary facilities are more sensitive to the financial incentives to screen out the most costly patients.

All of these findings should be interpreted with caution. First, most of the comparisons reported above do not control for many of the factors other than ownership that can affect institutional policies. Second, there is considerable variation in the behavior of health care organizations within any ownership category. Among investor-owned institutions, undoubtedly many discriminate less than the average nonprofit facility. Wise policymakers will take this variation into account. Third, before reacting to ownership-related differences, such as access restrictions imposed by for-profit providers, policymakers should, however, understand the origins of those screening practices. Like all health institutions, for-profit facilities respond to prevailing financial incentives. If they differ from nonproprietary providers in this respect, it is because they seem to respond more vigorously to those incentives. The existence of large numbers of inadequately insured or uninsured citizens in this country creates incentives for all health institutions to screen patients on the basis of ability to pay. For-profit institutions are more likely to do so, but as the data presented above reveal, private nonprofit facilities also restrict access far more than do public health care providers.

Prospective-payment systems, like Medicare's DRGs, are specifically designed to encourage facilities to specialize in the care they deliver and thus to choose carefully the patients they treat (Comptroller General 1980, 34–62). Hospitals are free, under this prospective-payment system, to "specialize" in the care of low-cost, uncomplicated patients. Indeed, all facilities, whatever their form of ownership, will benefit economically by specializing to some degree in treating such relatively profitable patients, and screening on the basis of cost will almost certainly increase among nonprofit facilities. Here too, however, investor-owned facilities seem likely to respond to these economic incentives more vigorously than will other providers.

The greater responsiveness of for-profit providers to financial incentives can be an asset as well as a liability. From the mid-1950s through the mid-1970s, many policy initiatives sought to encourage the expansion of the industry. The investor-owned sector responded most vigorously (Schlesinger 1985; Vladeck 1980, 250), as the history of Medicare's end-stage renal disease (ESRD) program illustrates. The 1972 ESRD amendments to the Social Security Act were intended to assure unrestricted access to care for all those with renal failure. The for-profit sector reacted more rapidly to the economic opportunity created by this new entitlement, opening facilities in many communities that were disproportionately poor or populated by minorities, areas in which nonprofit providers had been unable or unwilling to operate (Plough et al. 1984; Lowrie & Hampers 1982, 191–204).

Policymakers should recognize, therefore, that the screening practices of for-profit health facilities result in no small measure from overt public policy decisions or from the failure of American government to alleviate some major social problems. The growth of proprietary institutions highlights that we have no clear policy toward, nor consensus about, what constitutes adequate access to medical care for our citizens. Nor is there any agreement on the responsibility of medical providers either to individuals seeking care or to the community in which providers are located.

While we struggle to reach a consensus, the spread of proprietary health care will exact a price. Prospective-payment systems and increased reliance on for-profit institutions may threaten the viability of government-owned facilities (E. Brown 1983; Lewin & Lewin 1984, 9). In the hospital sector, for example, private providers will find it profitable to avoid costly patients within any particular DRG category. These patients will be channeled to public institutions (Feder, Hadley, & Mullner 1984). For any particular DRG, then, costs in public institutions will grow over time, creating the impression that they are less efficient compared to the private sector. This will undoubtedly lead to pressures to close more public hospitals, further exacerbating restrictions on access. Local, state, and federal governments must face the need to protect the financial stability of these facilities, which, in many areas, ensure only a minimum level of access to medical care.

Over the long term, the rise of proprietary institutions will magnify the effect of prevailing incentives to discriminate against patients who are unable to pay for their care or whose treatment is particularly costly. As disparities in access to care among different groups of citizens become more glaring, American society may be driven sooner than it might otherwise have been into providing all citizens with protection against the cost of illness. It would be ironic if the spread of for-profit medicine created conditions that prompted massive new governmental interventions into the organization and financing of American medicine. It would be a further irony if private nonprofit institutions, in responding to the competitive challenge of proprietary chains, helped create these very same conditions on a scale much larger than the proprietary sector alone could produce.

CONCLUSION AND DISCUSSION

Three points are central to any discussion about nonprofits and American medical care. The first is that factors other than the legal form of organization—whether nonprofit, profit, or governmental—have dominated the shape of American medicine and still do. To date, who pays for whose health care and how, the number and distribution of physicians and nurses, the organizational characteristics of payers and providers, and the larger political and economic environment—all these factors dwarf changes in corporate form in giving shape to how doctors, patients, and health insurance interact.

Second, legal forms often are held to stand for other institutional features associated with but not identical to the nonprofit, profit, or governmental structure of ownership. The most prominent dispute of the 1980s—inaccurately labeled as the rise of profit-making firms in health—in fact stood for several developments. It represented in part medical capitalism in the form of large-scale corporate investment in medicine (as with HCA and AHS) (Goldsmith 1984, 15). It stood as well for a spirit of entrepreneurialism—to use one of the vulgarities—that denoted a newer orientation toward profit, innovation, marketing sensitivity, and the like (New York Academy of Medicine 1985). And, finally, it stood for the scale and geographic reach of new hospital units—religious, profit making, or nonprofit—that range over many sites (chains) and may, as has HCA, vertically integrate with drug suppliers, insurance firms, or hospital product firms.

Our third point arises from the evidence on comparative performance set out above. Although we have emphasized the confusion and overstatement about the importance of ownership forms in medicine, there do appear to be systematic, ownership-related differences in the practices of health institutions. It thus seems reasonable to consider such differences as the basis for some public policies in the health industry.

Putting the Profit-Nonprofit Distinction in Perspective

A simple thought experiment brings out the first point of this conclusion. But consider first the reasonable and widely held view that American medicine has, for the last 30 years, been in considerable difficulty.

Access to adequate care remains a serious problem for millions despite the growth of private insurance and Medicare and Medicaid. Although figures vary considerably, at least 20 million people in the 1980s were without insurance coverage at all, private or public. Another 10 percent of the population—some 22 million in 1980—had inadequate protection against the most substantial medical expenditures—hospitalization and physician services (Munnell 1986). And another 20 percent lacked insurance against catastrophic expenses beyond 15 percent of annual income (Heineman 1985; Davis 1985; Marmor & Dunham 1985).

The *costs of care*—however financed—inflated enormously, rising from some $70 billion in 1970 to more than $400 billion in 1985 without commensurate improvements in quality or utilization.[26] And finally, there was widespread concern that insurance costs and greater pressure for cost reduction threatened further the quality of care available to Americans when they get it.

The simple thought experiment is this: if one imagines removing all the more recent developments in organizational forms—the growth of chains and profit-making hospitals—would any serious analyst of American medicine doubt that the above critique would remain substantially correct? We think the answer is no, one would not.

The continuing problems with access and costs point to the presence of fundamental, long-standing features of American medicine that only partially manifest themselves in the overheated debate about the proper legal form of organization.

Clarifying the Real Changes in American Medical Care

The growth of investor-owned health care facilities, for example, has been viewed by proponents as the elixir for all that ails the American health care system. Opponents see it as indicative of the virtual abandonment of a set of cherished social institutions and values. Both sides view the growth of the for-profit sector as foreshadowing a systemwide transformation of the health industry—and perhaps its complete conversion to proprietary auspices.

In fact, it seemed unlikely in the 1980s that such radical changes would occur. As we have seen, there have historically been a number of pronounced shifts in the relative importance of nonprofit and for-profit health care providers. These will continue to occur in the future in response to changes in private wants and in public subsidies, the changing authority of medical professionals, and the introduction of new technologies and services.

Whatever the history of the nonprofit in American medicine, the evidence of its performance, relatively speaking, does not clearly support either side of the nonprofit or for-profit debate. What is clear is that there has been a massive shift in the *character* of American medicine, not a shift in the dominant *form*. The growth of the for-profit chains, the challenge to business-as-usual, and the consequent shifts in the behavior of nonprofits are missed if one concentrates on nonprofit market share alone. If anything, the infusion of new capital in medicine has promoted competitive behavior in the industry, further exacerbating and, at the same time, obscuring the very conditions that should be the central subject of debate, namely, access and cost.

The Policy Implications of Differences in Nonprofit and For-Profit Health Institutions

We discussed above those differences and similarities revealed by the social science literature. We did not ask the question of to whom these differences would be important. Judging from the past behavior of nonprofit and for-profit health agencies, it seems inappropriate to simplistically relate ownership form to the achievement of socially valued goals. Both for-profit and nonprofit health care providers have, in different ways, served important public goals. The entry of for-profit providers has made available services that otherwise would have been too limited to meet rapidly growing or shifting patterns of utilization. The nonprofit form has provided a medium for innovative delivery of services and has provided, and continues in many instances to provide, an important source of care for those without the means (or insurance) to finance care.

Eliminating one form of ownership would neither obviate nor render catastrophically large existing policy problems, such as ensuring the availability of health services at reasonable cost and quality.[27] Although shifts in ownership are clearly neither the source of nor the solution to current failings of American medical care, the observed differences between nonprofit and for-profit performance are relevant to health policy. When health care as of 1993 costs $900 billion annually, the possibility of cutting costs by even 10 percent through shifting services to the most efficient providers is attractive. In a system, however, in which a large portion of consumers remain abysmally uninformed about their options for treatment and the quality of the care they receive, the threat of cutting quality in the pursuit of providers' self-interest is a real and important concern.

Similarly, although there exist cost differences of up to 10 percent between for-profit and nonprofit providers—the former higher for some services, the latter for others—prohibiting one form of ownership from offering services would have only a small effect on the spiraling inflation of medical costs.

To summarize our conclusions, there do not seem to be appreciable differences for most American patients in the care provided by for-profit and nonprofit hospitals. We are not saying no differences exist—indeed, we document them—but we want rather to emphasize that the near-term effects of the loss of market share by nonprofit hospitals are not associated with the dire predictions of the critics.

Ownership and Directions for Future Health Policies

If one shifts the question slightly, however, our interpretation changes substantially. There appear to be large differences between the forms of ownership and management for medical care entrepreneurs, who want to take profits out of medical care in the form of stock ownership (and are big winners), and for doctors, who have been profit makers all along but are losing control to new profit takers.

It is unclear, given that doctors and other medical personnel have been making the functional equivalent of profits—and high ones indeed under the old regime—whether the total amount of profit and the level of cost will go up under the altered regime.[28] Who will benefit, however, and who will be accountable to whom, will change. To state it briefly, the small entrepreneurs—particularly physicians—seem to be losing power to the larger organized corporate institutions exemplified by Humana and Hospital Corporation of America and, in part, by the new nonprofit systems. Some of the changes occurring, particularly the vertical and horizontal integration of medical care facilities, are historically unprecedented in health. Yet this is a familiar stage in the development of Western capitalism—the displacement of smaller units by larger ones in the name of rationalization.[29]

The argument, therefore, is not solely over profits or profit making. It is over the *control* of patients, profits, and professional privilege. The argument is not so much about organizational forms as about the incremental decline of a service ethos—more naked in one sector, more camouflaged in the other. The culture of American medicine, already entrepreneurial and commercial by international comparison, will probably grow more so (Marmor & Klein 1986).

All one needs to add here are the memorable words of the executive vice president of American Medical International, who laid out the full view that medicine is nothing but an ordinary market service. In explaining why hospitals are justified in getting tough with patients who cannot pay for care, Bruce Andrews noted that "we don't expect Safeway and A&P to give away free food for people who can't afford it." This casual remark—and especially its casual dismissal of centuries of concern that the care of the sick imposes special obligations on both the givers of care and the community as a whole—is terribly revealing. Of equal concern is the behavior of the religiously affiliated institution that carefully nurtures its sponsorship in its public relations while sending certain cases down the road to the local county hospital.[30] The relative triumph of commercialism and the long decline of professional authority mark contemporary American medicine, not particular forms within it.

The central place of nonprofits in American medicine had been, for some fifty years, largely unchallenged. The community hospital—nonprofit in form, local in roots, often religious in character, with physicians permitted to use its capital as they brought in patients—was ubiquitous, an American institution that by the 1950s had the quality of the familiar, the taken-for-granted. As the problem of medical inflation became epidemic in the late 1960s and 1970s, that form, along with much else in American medicine, was increasingly criticized, challenged, and sometimes even ridiculed.

The typical challenge was to point out the gap between the mission of the nonprofit and the reality, the ever-increasing revenues bargained for by insurance companies, governments, and patients with the zeal often associated with capitalist enterprise. For much of the postwar period, this critique was associated with the alternative of government regulation and, for some, with the dream of national health insurance. But by the end of the 1970s, a wholly different alternative had emerged from this common diagnosis. It was that competition—from health maintenance organizations and then from the chains of profit-making hospitals—would right the wrongs of medicine. Increased competition, it was argued, would help us all, and the pressure of profit seeking and the vaunted efficiencies of that for-profit model of corporate organizations were widely touted (Marmor, Boyer, & Greenberg 1983). It is this fight that has set the context for our discussion of the role of nonprofits in medicine.

The vices of the for-profits do not exonerate the nonprofits, although one could hardly tell from the high-minded preachiness of some in the nonprofit health world (Relman 1980). Nor does the inflationary history of the nonprofit health institutions make the proprietary institutions an answer to the costliness of American medicine. There are limits to what can be said by distinguishing among organizational forms; the differences are simply not that great. But there should be few limits to the vigilance with which we examine all health institutions and apply the appropriate constraints to the vices of their organizational virtues. There may be some areas where the innovative, energetic pursuit of profit will, under the right rules, bring social gain. Drug production and laboratory medicine now operate under such rules, with ambiguous results (Evans 1984, 209–31). More competition between providers will almost certainly bring increased sensitivity to patients (particularly well-insured ones) and the costs of their care. Whether that sensitivity will mean caring or coddling is uncertain. And whether the concern about costs will produce true efficiency gains is uncertain, but possible (Evans 1984, 225–26).

There are parallel considerations for the nonprofits in health. Will the patient screening that is now more profitable produce a reaction, particularly among physicians and nurses? Will the nonprofit rationale—

the commitment to caring for the sick, however financed—reenter our debates in such a way that responsible action is fiscally rewarded or, at the very least, not penalized? Will physicians discover anew the advantages of the nonprofit form without our policymakers losing the distinction between autonomy that helps patients and independence that simply increases physician incomes (Majone 1984)? Will we, in short, recognize that health care has been, for very good reasons, a not-only-for-profit industry and that no amount of marketing hype will make vulnerable patients the wary consumers of Adam Smith's theoretical markets?

The challenge for public policy will be to discover rules of the medical game that constrain the vices of both rampant commercialism and complacent professionalism. The real uncertainty is whether our polity is capable of such sophistication.

REFERENCES

American Hospital Association. 1983. *Hospital Statistics*. Chicago: American Hospital Association.

Arrow, Kenneth. 1963. "Uncertainty and the Welfare Economics of Medical Care." *American Economic Review* 53, no. 5:941–73.

Bays, Carson. 1979. "Cost Comparisons for For-Profit and Nonprofit Hospitals." *Social Science and Medicine* 13:219–27.

———. 1983a. "Patterns of Hospital Growth: The Case of Profit Hospitals." *Medical Care* 21:950–57.

———. 1983b. "Why Most Private Hospitals Are Nonprofit." *Journal of Policy Analysis and Management* 2:367.

Bishop, C. 1980. "Nursing Home Cost Studies and Reimbursement Issues." *Health Care Financing Review* 2 (Spring):47–64.

Brown, E. 1983. "Public Hospitals on the Brink: Their Problems and Their Options." *Journal of Health Politics, Policy and Law* 7, no. 4 (Winter):927–44.

Brown, Lawrence D. 1983. *Politics and Health Care Organizations: HMOs as Federal Policy*. Washington, D.C.: Brookings.

———. 1985. "Technocratic Corporatism and Administrative Reform in Medicare." *Journal of Health Politics, Policy, and Law,* 10, no. 3 (Fall):579–99.

———. 1986. "The Proper Boundaries of the Role of Government." *Bulletin of the New York Academy of Medicine* 62, no. 1 (January–February):15.

Caswell, R., and Cleverly, W. 1983. "Cost Analysis of the Ohio Nursing Home Industry." *Health Services Research* 18 (Fall):359–82.

Clark, Robert C. 1980. "Does the Nonprofit Form Fit the Hospital Industry?" *Harvard Law Review* 93, no. 7 (May):1416.

Clarkson, Kenneth. 1972. "Some Implications of Property Rights in Hospital Man-
     agement." *Journal of Law and Economics* 15:363.
Comptroller General of the United States. 1980. *Rising Hospital Costs Can be
     Restrained by Regulating Payments and Improving Management.* Publi-
     cation no. HRD-80-72. Washington, D.C.: U.S. Government Printing Of-
     fice.
Cromwell, J., and Kanak, J. R. 1982. "The Effects of Prospective Reimbursement
     Programs on Hospital Adoption and Service Sharing." *Health Care Fi-
     nancing Review* 4, no. 2:67–88.
Danzon, P. 1982. "Hospital 'Profits': The Effects of Reimbursement Policies."
     Journal of Health Economics 1 (May):29–52.
Davis, Karen. 1985. "Access to Health Care: A Matter of Fairness." In Center for
     National Policy, *Health Care: How to Improve It and Pay for It.* Wash-
     ington, D.C.: Center for National Policy.
Drake, D. 1980. "The Cost of Hospital Regulation." In A. Levin, ed., *Regulating
     Health Care: The Struggle for Control (Proceedings of the Academy of
     Political Science* 33, no. 4:45–59).
Dunham, Andrew; Morone, James; and White, William. 1982. "Restoring Medical
     Markets: Implications for the Poor." *Journal of Health Politics, Policy
     and Law* 7, no. 2 (Summer):488–501.
Eisenberg, Leon. 1985. "The Right to Health Care: For Patients or For-Profits."
     Paper presented at the annual meeting of the American Psychiatric Asso-
     ciation, Dallas, Texas, May 21.
Enthoven, Alain. 1980. *Health Plan: The Only Practical Solution to the Soaring
     Costs of Health Care.* Reading, Mass.: Addison-Wesley.
Ermann, D., and Gabel, J. 1984. "Multihospital Systems: Issues and Empirical
     Findings." *Health Affairs* 3, no. 1:50–64.
Evans, Robert G. 1984. *Strained Mercy: The Economics of Canadian Health
     Care.* Toronto: Butterworth.
Feder, Judith M. 1977. *Medicare: The Politics of Federal Hospital Insurance.*
     Lexington, Mass.: Lexington Books.
Feder, Judith, and Hadley, Jack. 1985. "The Economically Unattractive Patient:
     Who Cares?" *Bulletin of the New York Academy of Medicine* 61, no. 1
     (January–February):68–75.
Feder, J.; Hadley, J.; and Mullner, R. 1984. "Falling through the Cracks: Poverty,
     Insurance Coverage, and Hospital Care for the Poor, 1980 and 1982."
     Milbank Memorial Fund Quarterly 62 (Fall):544–66.
Feldstein, P. 1978. *Health Associations and the Demand for Legislation.* Cam-
     bridge, Mass.: Ballinger.
Fox, Daniel. 1986. "The Consequences of Consensus: American Health Policy in
     the Twentieth Century," *Milbank Memorial Fund Quarterly* 64, no. 1:76–
     99.
Frech, H. E. 1976. "The Property Rights Theory of the Firm: Empirical Results
     from a Natural Experiment." *Journal of Political Economy* 84:143–52.

Frech, H., and Ginsberg, P. 1981. "The Cost of Nursing Home Care in the United States: Government Ownership, Financing, and Efficiency." In J. Van Der Gaag and M. Perlman, eds., *Health, Economics, and Health Economics*. New York: North-Holland.

Freeland, Mark S., and Schendler, Carol E. 1984. "Health Spending in the 1980's." *Health Care Financing Review* 5 (Spring):7.

Gabel, John, and Ermann, Dan. 1985. "Preferred Provider Organizations: Performance, Problems, and Promise." *Health Affairs* 4:24–40.

Gage, Larry S. 1985. "Impact on the Public Hospitals." *Bulletin of the New York Academy of Medicine* 61, no. 1 (January–February):75–81.

Gardner, K. 1981. "Profit and the End-Stage Renal Disease Program." *New England Journal of Medicine* 305:461–62.

Goldberg, V. 1975. "Some Emerging Problems of Prepaid Health Plans in the Medi-Cal System." *Policy Analysis* 1 (Winter):55–68.

Goldsmith, Jeffrey. 1984. "Death of a Paradigm: The Challenge of Competition." *Health Affairs* (Fall):7–19.

Grady, Denise. 1986. "The Cruel Price of Cutting Medical Expenses." *Discover* 7, no. 5 (May):25–43.

Gray, Bradford H. 1985. "Overview: Origins and Trends." *Bulletin of the New York Academy of Medicine* 61, no. 1 (January–February):7–23.

Gray, Bradford H., ed. 1983. *The New Health Care for Profit: Doctors and Hospitals in a Competitive Environment*. Washington, D.C.: National Academy Press.

Hansmann, Henry. 1980. "The Role of Non-profit Enterprise." *Yale Law Journal* 89, no. 5 (April):835–901.

"Health Care Costs to Hit 12% of Gross National Product: Study." 1984. *Hospital Week* 20, no. 33 (August 17):2.

Heineman, B. W., Jr. 1985. "Introduction: Health Policy and Health Politics." In Center for National Policy, *Health Care: How to Improve It and Pay for It*. Washington, D.C.: Center for National Policy.

Held, P., and Pauly, M. 1982. "An Economic Analysis of the Production and Cost of Renal Dialysis Treatments." Working Paper 3064–03. Washington, D.C.: Urban Institute.

Holmberg, R., and Anderson, N. 1968. "Implications of Ownership for Nursing Home Care." *Medical Care* 6 (July–August):300–7.

Homer, C. G.; Gradham, D. D.; and Rushefsky, M. 1984. "Investor-Owned and Not-for-profit Hospitals: Beyond the Cost and Revenue Debate." *Health Affairs* 3, no. 1:133–36.

Horty, John F., and Mulholland, Daniel M. 1983. "Legal Differences between Investor-Owned and Nonprofit Health Care Institutions." In Bradford Gray, ed., *The New Health Care for Profit: Doctors and Hospitals in a Competitive Environment*. Washington, D.C.: National Academy Press.

Koetting, M. 1980. *Nursing-Home Organization and Efficiency*. Lexington, Mass.: Lexington Books.

Koten, John. 1985. "Baxter to Buy American Hospital Supply." *Wall Street Journal*, July 16, p. 2.

Koten, John, and Waldholz, Michael. 1985. "Baxter Travenol Bids $3.6 Billion for Supply Firm." *Wall Street Journal*, June 24, p. 2.

Krizay, J., and Wilson, A. 1974. *The Patient as Consumer*. Lexington, Mass.: Lexington Books.

Kushman, J. E., and Nuckton, C. F. 1977. "Further Evidence on the Relative Performance of Proprietary and Nonprofit Hospitals." *Medical Care* 15, no. 3:189–204.

Lave, J., and Lave, J. 1974. *The Hospital Construction Act*. Washington, D.C.: American Enterprise Institute.

Law, Sylvia. 1974. *Blue Cross: What Went Wrong?* New Haven: Yale University Press.

Lewin, Lawrence S.; Derzon, Robert A.; and Margulies, Rhea. 1981. "Investor-Owneds and Nonprofits Differ in Economic Performance." *Hospitals* (July):52–58.

Lewin, M. E., and Lewin, L. S. 1984. "Health Care for the Uninsured." *Business Health* 1, no. 9:9–14.

Lowrie, E. G. 1981. "Treatment of End-Stage Renal Disease." *New England Journal of Medicine* 304:356.

Lowrie, E. G., and Hampers, C. L. 1982. "Proprietary Dialysis and the End-Stage Renal Disease Program." *Dialysis and Transplant* 11:191–204.

Luft, Harold. 1981. *Health Maintenance Organizations: Dimensions of Performance*. New York: Wiley.

Majone, G. 1984. "Professionalism and Nonprofit Organizations." *Journal of Health Politics, Policy, and Law* 8, no. 4 (Winter)639–59.

Marmor, Theodore R. 1973. *The Politics of Medicare*. Chicago: Aldine.

———. 1983. *Political Analysis and American Medical Care*. Cambridge: Cambridge University Press.

Marmor, Theodore R., and Dunham, Andrew. 1985. "The Politics of Health Policy Reform: Origins, Alternatives, and a Possible Prescription." In Center for National Policy, *Health Care: How to Improve It and Pay for It*. Washington, D.C.: Center for National Policy.

Marmor, T. R., and Klein, R. 1986. "Cost vs. Care," *Health Matrix* 4, no. 1 (Spring):19–24.

Marmor, Theodore R.; Boyer, Richard; and Greenberg, Julie. 1983. "Medical Care and Procompetitive Reform." In Theodore R. Marmor, *Political Analysis and American Medical Care*. Cambridge: Cambridge University Press.

Marmor, Theodore R.; Wittman, Donald A.; and Heagy, Thomas C. 1983. "The Politics of Medical Inflation." In Theodore R. Marmor, *Political Analysis and American Medical Care*. Cambridge: Cambridge University Press.

Marsh, Frank H. 1985. "Health Care Cost Containment and the Duty to Treat." *Journal of Legal Medicine* 6 (June):157–90.

Morone, James. 1985. "The Unruly Rise of Medical Capitalism." *Hasting Center Report* (August):4–31.

Morone, James, and Dunham, Andrew. 1985. "Slouching towards National Health Insurance: The New Health Care Politics." *Yale Journal on Regulation* 2:263.

Morone, James, and Marmor, Theodore. 1983. "Representing Consumer Interests: The Case of American Health Planning." In Theodore R. Marmor, *Political Analysis and American Medical Care*. Cambridge: Cambridge University Press.

Mullner, Ross, and Hadley, Jack. 1984. "Interstate Variations in the Growth of Chain-Operated Proprietary Hospitals, 1973–82." *Inquiry* 21:144–57.

Munnell, Alicia. 1986. "Ensuring Entitlement to Health Care Services." *Bulletin of the New York Academy of Medicine* 62, no. 1 (January–February):61–74.

Neuhauser, D. 1974. "The Future of Proprietaries in American Health Services." In C. C. Havighurst, ed., *Regulating Health Facilities Construction*. Washington, D.C.: American Enterprise Institute.

New York Academy of Medicine. 1985. "The New Entrepreneurialism in Health Care: 1984 Annual Conference, New York Academy of Medicine." In *Bulletin of the New York Academy of Medicine* 61, no. 1 (January–February).

Nielsen, W. 1979. *The Endangered Sector*. New York: Columbia University Press.

Nutter, D. O. 1984. "Access to Care and the Evolution of Corporate, For-Profit Medicine." *New England Journal of Medicine* 311:917–19.

Pattison, R. V., and Katz, H. M. 1983. "Investor-Owned and Not-for-Profit Hospitals: A Comparison Based on California Data." *New England Journal of Medicine* 309:347–53.

Plough, A. L.; Salem, S. R.; Schwartz, M.; Weller, J. M.; and Ferguson, C. W. 1984. "Case Mix in End-Stage Renal Disease: Differences between Patients in Hospital-Based and Free-Standing Facilities." *New England Journal of Medicine* 310:1432–36.

Raffel, M. W. 1980. *The U.S. Health Care System: Origins and Functions*. New York: John Wiley.

Relman, Arnold S. 1980. "The New Medical Industrial Complex." *New England Journal of Medicine*. 303:963–70.

———. 1983. "Investor-Owned Hospitals and Health-Care Costs." *New England Journal of Medicine* 309:370.

Relman, A. S., and Rennie, D. 1980. "Treatment of End-Stage Renal Disease: Free but Not Equal." *New England Journal of Medicine* 303:996.

Riportella-Mueller, R., and Slesinger, D. 1982. "The Relationship of Ownership and Size to Quality of Care in Wisconsin Nursing Homes." *Gerontologist* 22 (Winter):429–34.

Rorem, R. 1939. "Enabling Legislation for Non-Profit Hospital Service Plans." *Law and Contemporary Problems* 6:528.

Rosenblatt, Rand E. 1978. "Health Care Reform and Administrative Law: A Structural Appraisal." *Yale Law Journal* 88, no. 2 (December):243–336.

Ruchlin, Hirsch S. 1979. "An Analysis of Regulatory Issues and Options in Long-Term Care." In V. LaPorte and J. Rubin, eds., *Reform and Regulation in Long-Term Care*. New York: Praeger.

Salamon, Lester M., and Abramson, Alan J. 1982. *The Federal Budget and the Nonprofit Sector*. Washington, D.C.: Urban Institute.

Schlenker, R. E., and Shaughnessy, P. W. 1984. "Case Mix, Quality, and Cost Relationships in Colorado Nursing Homes." *Health Care Financing Review* 61:6.

Schlesinger, M. 1984. "Public, For-Profit, and Private Nonprofit Enterprises." Doctoral dissertation.

———. 1985. "The Rise of Proprietary Health Care." *Business Health* 2, no. 1:7–12.

Schlesinger, M., and Blumenthal, D. 1986. "Ownership and Access to Health Care: New Evidence and Policy Implications." Unpublished.

Schlesinger, M., and Dorwart, R. 1984. "Ownership and Mental Health Services: A Reappraisal." *New England Journal of Medicine* 311:959–65.

Schlesinger, M.; Blumenthal, D.; and Schlesinger, E. 1986. "Profits under Pressure: The Economic Performance of Investor-Owned and Nonprofit Health Maintenance Organizations." *Medical Care* 24:615–27.

Sherman, H. David, and Chilingerian, Jon A. 1984. "For-Profit vs. Nonprofit Hospitals: The Effect of the Profit Motive on the Management of Operations." Unpublished.

Shortell, S.; Morrison, E.; Hughes, S.; and Coverdill, J. 1986. "The Impact of Multi-Institutional Systems on Service Provision." In L. Rossiter, R. Scheffler, G. Wilensky, and N. McCall, eds., *Advances in Health Economics and Health Services Research,* vol. 7. Greenwich, Conn.: JAI Press.

Silver, L. H. 1974. "The Legal Accountability of Nonprofit Hospitals." In C. C. Havighurst, ed., *Regulating Health Facilities Construction*. Washington, D.C.: American Enterprise Institute.

Sloan, F. A., and Becker, E. R. 1984. "Cross-Subsidies and Payment for Hospital Care." *Journal of Health Politics, Policy, and Law* 8, no. 4 (Winter):660–85.

Sloan, F. A., and Vraciu, R. A. 1983. "Investor-Owned and Not-for-Profit Hospitals: Addressing Some Issues." *Health Affairs* 2, no. 1:25–37.

Smith, D. 1981. *Long-Term Care in Transition: The Regulation of Nursing Homes*. Washington, D.C.: AUPHA Press.

Stanford Law Review. 1962. "Recent Development: Private Hospital Must Admit Unmistakable Emergency Cases." *Stanford Law Review* 14, no. 4 (July):910–18.

Starr, Paul. 1982. *The Social Transformation of American Medicine*. New York: Basic Books.

Starr, Paul, and Marmor, Theodore. 1984. "The U.S.: A Social Forecast." In Jean
    de Kervasdoué, John R. Kimberly, and Victor G. Rodwin, *The End of
    an Illusion*. Berkeley: University of California Press.
Steinwald, B., and Neuhauser, D. 1970. "The Role of the Proprietary Hospital."
    Journal of Law and Contemporary Problems 35:817–38.
Stevens, R. 1971. *American Medicine and the Public Interest*. New Haven: Yale
    University Press.
———. 1982. "'A Poor Sort of Memory': Voluntary Hospitals and Government
    before the Depression." *Milbank Memorial Fund Quarterly* 60 (Fall):551–
    84.
Stevens, R., and Stevens, R. 1974. *Welfare Medicine in America*. New York: Free
    Press.
Titmuss, R. 1971. *The Gift Relationship*. New York: Vintage Books.
Ullman, S. 1983. "Ownership and Performance in the Long-Term Health Care In-
    dustry." University of Miami, Department of Economics Working Paper.
Vladeck, B. C. 1980. *Unloving Care*. New York: Basic Books.
Waldholz, Michael. 1985. "American Hospital Plans to Merge with Hospital Corp.
    in Stock Swap." *Wall Street Journal*, April 1, p. 3.
Weisbrod, B. C., and Schlesinger, M. 1981. "Benefit-Cost Analysis in the Mental
    Health Area: Issues and Directions for Research." In *Economics and
    Mental Health*. National Institute of Mental Health Series EN no. 1,
    DHHS Publication no. (ADM)81–1114. Washington, D.C.: U.S. Govern-
    ment Printing Office, 8–28.
Weller, Charles D. 1984. "Free Choice as a Restraint of Trade in American Health
    Care Delivery and Insurance." *Iowa Law Review* 69, no. 5 (July):1351–
    92.
Yordy, Karl D. 1986. "Current and Future Developments in Health Care." *Bulletin
    of the New York Academy of Medicine* 62, no. 1:27–38.

Chapter 5
Cutting Waste by Making Rules: Promises, Pitfalls, and Realistic Prospects

WITH JAN BLUSTEIN

American medical costs, one hardly needs to say, continue to rise relentlessly. In 1990, health expenditures consumed approximately 12.2 percent of America's Gross National Product (GNP).[1] A decade earlier, the share was 9.1 percent.[2] In 1970, we spent approximately 7.4 percent.[3] There has developed an apparent consensus—among government, labor, and profession leaders—that costs must be contained. At the same time, there is widespread agreement that access must be universalized. As a result, many believe that excruciatingly hard choices are unavoidable.

This perceived dilemma has led to a great deal of talk about rationing.[4] The tenor of the commentary indicates that it is a fearsome solution to our present troubles—painful and divisive, entailing choices that no one wants to make but which must be faced due to inescapable scarcity.[5] Both contemporary rhetoric and current health policy, however, hold

From *University of Pennsylvania Law Review*, Vol. 140, No. 5 (May 1992), pp. 1543–72. Reprinted by permission.

Jan Blustein was supported by a National Research Scientist Award from the Agency for Health Care Policy and Research; Theodore Marmor received support from the Canadian Institute for Advanced Research, of which he is a fellow. The authors thank David Willis, Philip Lee, Victor Rodwin, and Colin Dayan for their helpful comments.

out the hope of a far more agreeable alternative. Galvanized by the realization that much medical care is of uncertain value, and bolstered by findings that show significant variation in medical practice patterns, a coalition of policymakers, politicians, and researchers is now actively engaged in seeking to contain costs by eliminating wasteful care. This appears an attractive course. Waste cutting, unlike rationing, does not connote the cruel denial of necessary care. On the contrary, it suggests saving people from medical interventions that would not have done them any good. If "rationing" is the fearsome alternative, "cutting waste" is the benign one.

While consensus grows that wasteful practice is a problem, there is considerable disagreement about the solution. Such disagreement is hardly surprising, since cutting waste is merely a goal, not a program. Cutting waste can mean any of a number of things. It can mean regionalizing services, instituting yearly expenditure targets, implementing managed care systems, or developing elaborate review mechanisms to constrain the diffusion of new technologies. Indeed, the idea of "cutting waste" is so broad in its potential scope that it can subsume many hotly debated reforms in the field of health policy. Like Health Maintenance Organizations, competition, and Diagnostic Related Groups before it, it is another vaunted panacea, the new great answer to arrive on the American health policy agenda.[6]

This chapter critically assesses the widely advertised plan to cut waste by making microallocational rules for the provision of medical care. Such rules, variously denominated "practice parameters,"[7] "clinical guidelines,"[8] and "standards of care,"[9] are aimed at ensuring that no patient is subjected to "wasteful" care by specifying what treatments particular patients should receive. For example, the rule that "healthy patients under 40 years of age without a family history of heart disease should not be given an electrocardiogram" is a practice parameter. It could be used by physicians to guide day-to-day treatment decisions. It could also be used by payers to control reimbursement, and by policymakers to appraise aggregate data about medical care utilization.[10]

Our analysis raises the fundamental but too-little-discussed question of what constitutes waste. Our central claim is that so-called wasteful practice is a conceptual hodgepodge, which encompasses treatments that are (1) ineffective; (2) of uncertain effectiveness; (3) ethically troubling; or (4) not allocationally efficient.[11] From this starting point, we address issues of rulemaking and resource allocation and ask the following questions: Can all four of these types of wasteful care be identified in ways that are scientifically defensible and administratively practicable? What obstacles must be faced to make cutting waste by making rules into a *policy* in each case? Are there American institutions and attitudes that would make such rulemaking more costly, and therefore less attractive, than it seems? And can any (or all) of these four types of waste be cut without confronting the dilemma of difficult choices? But before approaching these questions, we begin by briefly reviewing the ways in which the problem of wasteful care has been framed by health care analysts, providers, and policymakers.

LOOSE TALK ABOUT "WASTE"

Terms like "wasteful," "ineffective," "inappropriate," "of unproven effectiveness," "unnecessary," and even "irrational" are used loosely and often interchangeably in the literature that is critical of current medical practice. Commentators have lamented the prevalence of unnecessary elective surgery,[12] gratuitous "little ticket" diagnostic tests,[13] and expensive treatments for AIDS patients.[14] It is tempting to assume that these practices share some fundamental characteristic that places them within a unified category of wasteful medical treatments.

Although the temptation is evident, assimilating various "inappropriate" types of care within the rhetoric of waste cutting is at best confusing. Take the example of the rules that determine when physician office visits are "medically necessary."[15] As one physician explained it:

> Medicare has set guidelines that for a given condition, you're only allowed to see patients so many times. That doesn't mean that you can't see them more often—you certainly can—but they won't pay for it. . . .
>
> It takes a great deal of time . . . because I have to explain to them why Medicare may not pay for their visit to me. You're legally obligated to explain to the patient that this is considered medically unnecessary. Well, that choice of words implies to most patients that you're giving poor medical care. You're making them come back too often. And I think it's terrible.
>
> It wastes 20 minutes of my time explaining to them that no, its not really medically unnecessary, that that's just how Medicare has chosen to word the new form.[16]

Making "expensive" synonymous with "medically unnecessary" seems a particularly troubling example of bureaucratically sanctioned linguistic drift. But it is not just linguistic territory that has been invaded

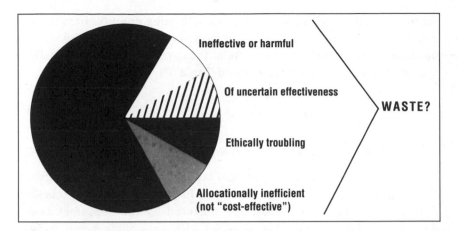

Figure 5.1 A problem for medical care cost containment.

by the waste cutters. Utilization review companies have moved beyond the realm of previewing surgical procedures and into the field of making allocational choices in the cases of very sick and dying patients. They employ "case managers" to direct the costly care of their sickest enrollees. This strategy can pay off handsomely. "Many cost-management companies are strengthening their 'case management' of patients who are seriously ill, with advanced cancer or AIDS, for example, or recovering from a stroke. 'The savings can average $10,000 to $15,000 per case and be as high as $400,000.'"[17] While some case managers may be truly well intentioned, intervening to help patients and save them from painful overtreatment, they also represent economic interests that will inevitably conflict at times with the interests of the patient. In the future, we are likely to hear more from case managers about "inappropriate," "ineffective," and "medically unnecessary" care. When we do, it will be hard to know exactly what this means. Is the proposed treatment harmful or worthless? Is it futile or just too costly?

These ambiguities must be faced in formulating a sensible strategy for controlling the cost of medical care in America. It would be enormously agreeable if cost containment could be achieved by cutting out a homogeneous wedge of present practices. But our analysis suggests that waste is heterogeneous (Figure 5.1), a claim worth exploring at some length. We need to know more about the four different types of waste. How prevalent are they? How do we determine that particular treatments fall into one of the four categories? What political, social, and professional obstacles will arise when standards are introduced forbidding wasteful practices? Will waste cutting erect barriers to beneficial care, or can waste cutting bypass such choices in medical care allocation? These four questions are at the core of the following section. Our main findings are summarized in Table 5.1.

A TAXONOMY OF "WASTE"

Ineffective (or Harmful) Treatment

Some Americans, expert and lay, believe that much of medical care is ineffective or positively harmful. In part a generalized rebellion against authority of the 1960s, and nurtured by the consumer health movement of the 1970s, this view found a passionate voice in Ivan Illich's 1976 book, *Medical Nemesis*.[18] His scathing critique of the medical profession's "poisons"[19] and "black magic"[20] never found widespread public acceptance. But the 1980s brought a wider condemnation of the medical profession. Today's conventional wisdom is that doctors have little idea of what they are doing.

> Consider what doctors, to say nothing of patients, don't know about the value of just one procedure. Every year about 80,000 Americans get a carotid endarterectomy, a kind of Roto-Rooter job on clogged neck arteries. Typically costing $9,000, counting the bill for a hospital stay, the operation is designed to prevent strokes. Another triumph of modern medicine? Or an overly risky, overdone alternative to cheaper drug therapy? Incredibly, no one knows for sure, and no one is tracking the patients on a systematic basis to find out.
>
> The same holds true for scores of other medical ministrations. Food companies know the impact of a redesigned ketchup bottle on sales. But the virtuosos performing hysterectomies, installing pacemakers and bypassing diseased coronary arteries have only patchy information about the real payoffs. "Half of what the medical profession does is of unverified effectiveness," asserts Dr. Paul M. Ellwood, Jr. of Minneapolis, [one] in a phalanx of physicians who want to cut down on the guesswork.[21]

Academic medicine is trying to answer this criticism. Researchers in a relatively new branch of investigation, clinical epidemiology, are trying to sort out which medical maneuvers are effective. Ideally, the research involves systematic and painstaking testing of therapies

Table 5.1
A taxonomy of wasteful care

Type of waste	Amount of waste	Issues in identifying waste	Costs of cutting waste by making rules	Does cutting waste mean denying benefit?
Ineffective of harmful	Unknown, since the effectiveness of most intervention is uncertain.	Requires an extensive scientific database. "Clinical judgment" introduces uncertainty.	Relatively few. Public probably will accept. Physicians have accepted the strategy (RAND/AMA cooperation). Entails administrative costs.	No.
Of uncertain effectiveness	Abundant, since the effectiveness of most interventions is uncertain.	See above.	Many. Physicians likely to resent intrusion on clinical judgment. Public unlikely to accept denial of care perceived to be beneficial.	Not known (hard choices).
Ethically troubling	Growing.	Requires an ethical consensus.	Many (need to distinguish between guidelines and rules to cut waste). Public discussion of rules to cut waste is controversial.	Perhaps (depends on values; hard choices).
Allocationally inefficient ("not cost-effective")	Unknown, since cost-benefit analysis and cost-effectiveness analysis work better in theory than in practice.	Requires the acquisition of scientific and economic data, as well as development of a consensus about values and an agreement about budgetary constraints.	Many. Rulemaking can be bitterly divisive. Public expects to get beneficial care regardless of costs. There may be legal obstacles to rulemaking. Physicians feel that consideration of costs taints professionalism.	Yes (hard choices).

through randomized controlled clinical trials. But these experiments, the "gold standard" for determining clinical effectiveness, are events of epic proportion, lasting for years, costing millions of dollars, involving thousands of patients, facing monumental bureaucratic barriers, and raising serious ethical issues.[22] Often, by the time clinical trials are completed, the technology they studied is outmoded.[23] Although other methodologies have been developed and can yield useful information,[24] physicians must regularly weigh the preponderance of imperfect evidence in order to estimate whether a particular patient might benefit from a particular intervention.[25] It is often possible to entertain some reasonable doubt (or to hold out some reasonable hope) that a treatment will be effective. While there is currently a great deal of enthusiasm about improving the scientific basis of medicine, and while there is surely room for improvement, a vast project to make medicine scientific can never keep up with innovations in medical practice. Nor is it likely to provide firm ground for determining correct choices in most clinical situations. Medical decision making is simply too complex.[26]

Given these limitations, how can ineffective treatments be identified? One approach is to augment imperfect information with the judgments of experts. Distinguished physicians, well versed in the scientific literature, can use their clinical judgment—their beliefs about what works, based on their own past practices—to produce estimates of effectiveness. And groups of physicians can combine their expert judgments to arrive at consensus. A group of researchers at the RAND Corporation has developed a method for generating this kind of professional consensus about what works (and what doesn't work) in medicine.[27] Because their innovative method has been so widely acclaimed and so often held up as a model for cutting waste by making rules, it warrants a brief review.

The RAND group's goal was to develop practice parameters for several widely used operations. They assembled a panel of distinguished physicians for each of the operations, and each panel member reviewed the available scientific literature about the procedure.[28] With a list of all of the possible clinical scenarios in which each procedure might be performed, each panelist made an assessment of the appropriateness of the intervention for each of the scenarios, based on the literature review and clinical judgment. After making independent assessments, the panel members met to discuss the cases and compare their ratings. They found there was substantial disagreement among them about the appropriateness of performing the operations in many clinical settings.[29] And so, after reviewing the cases together, the individual physicians rated each scenario again, and the revised ratings were combined into a group consensus rating of the appropriateness of treatment in each situation. For each clinical scenario, the surgery was rated as "appropriate," "inappropriate," or "equivocal." Inappropriate care was treatment in which "the expected health benefit[s] (i.e., increased life expectancy, relief of pain, reduction in anxiety, [and] improved functional capacity) [were] exceeded [by] the expected negative consequences (i.e., mortality, morbidity, anxiety of anticipating the procedure, pain produced by the procedure, and time lost from work)."[30] Roughly speaking, then, "inappropriate" was defined to mean ineffective or harmful.

The ratings have been used successfully in pilot programs to identify inappropriate care. Two prominent RAND researchers subsequently left the Santa Monica think tank to found Value Health Sciences, Inc., bringing along the RAND methodology. They then developed some innovative software that uses the expert consensus on appropriateness to deliver second opinions about physician's treatment choices. Value's clients employ utilization review nurses to quiz physicians about referrals for the selected procedures. Using Value's computer-driven questionnaire while talking over the telephone, the nurses gather information about prospective patients and then match each prospective patient to a previously rated clinical scenario. If the prior consensus suggested the operation was appropriate for that patient, the patient's insurance company pays for the hospital admission. If the rules identified the operation as inappropriate, the procedure is not covered. The referring physician may then appeal the decision regarding coverage with a doctor representing the utilization review company. In a trial run by the Aetna insurance company, 15 percent of 1,000 referrals for procedures were judged inappropriate; physicians appeals brought the number of actual refusals down to 9 percent.[31]

The successful implementation of the RAND/Value method is one of the first achievements of what has been called the "outcomes movement."[32] This informal coalition of academic researchers, government officials, physician professional organizations, and members of the health insurance industry has come together over several years in an effort to study what works in medicine, to define appropriate care, and to use that definition of appropriateness to eliminate allegedly wasteful care through the use of practice guidelines. While each participant has a slightly different sense of the movement's mission,[33] most share Paul Ellwood's ambitious vision:

> Outcomes management is a technology of patient experience
> designed to help patients, payers, and providers make rational
> medical care–related choices based on better insight into the
> effect of these choices on the patient's life. Outcomes man-
> agement consists of a . . . language of health outcomes; a
> national data base containing information and analysis on clin-
> ical, financial and health outcomes that estimates as best we
> can the relation between medical interventions and health out-
> comes, as well as the relation between health outcomes and
> money; and an opportunity for each decision-maker to have
> access to the analyses that are relevant to the choices they
> must make.[34]

Federal officials have been enthusiastic supporters of what has been
hailed—perhaps somewhat grandiosely—as "the third revolution in
health care."[35] Former Health Care Financing Administration (HCFA)
director William L. Roper, under pressure to contain Medicare's explosive growth, announced a major initiative to "evaluate and improve
medical practice" by using HCFA's mammoth databases to study the
outcomes of care given under that program.[36] In a related later development, the Department of Health and Human Services' National Center for Health Services Research (NCHSR) was renamed the Agency for
Health Care Policy and Research (AHCPR) and charged with "promoting
the quality, appropriateness, and effectiveness of health care" and di-
recting studies that would lead to the development of clinical guidelines
for "treatments or conditions that account for a significant portion of
Medicare expenditures."[37] With the new name came an increase in
federal funding. In 1991, the agency received over $60 million to inves-
tigate the outcomes of medical care and develop parameters to guide
clinical practice.[38] Three years earlier, as the NCHSR, the agency had
been given less than $2 million to support such efforts.[39] Many leaders
of private industry and health insurance firms are enthusiastic about
these developments, and foresee using the results to cut costs.[40]

The American Medical Association (AMA) is perhaps the least likely
of the coalition's members. Historically a staunch advocate of physician
autonomy, the AMA has teamed up with the RAND Corporation and the
Academic Medical Center Consortium, a group of major teaching hospitals,[41] to develop practice guidelines for use by "payers and utilization
and medical reviewers to define a range of practice options physicians
could use without incurring financial or other sanctions."[42] If the AMA's
embrace of the parameters initiative is somewhat puzzling—few phy-

sicians wish to do their patients harm, but none seem to want to be told what to do—organized medicine's position probably reflects the recognition that "if you can't beat em, join em." As AMA Executive Vice President James Todd explained, physicians must lead the effort to develop practice standards because they "can't afford to abdicate this responsibility to [the] bureaucratic computer screens of HCFA or commercial insurance companies."[43] Although support for the initiative must be viewed primarily as a kind of preemptive strike, practical parameters do offer some attractive features from the physicians' perspective.[44] First, they have a substantial educational potential. In a bewilderingly complex and rapidly changing technical environment, parameters can provide physicians with a simple, easily accessible reference guide. Second, in a hostile legal environment, adherence to "appropriate" practices may protect practitioners from malpractice liability.[45]

In summary, parameters *do* hold some promise in curbing ineffective or harmful care, and there is clearly energetic activity in support of their development. But the amount of time and money required to develop and implement the RAND/Value approach on a large scale, though unknown, is surely substantial. According to AHCPR officials, it has taken three years to move from the process of identifying conditions for guideline development to early pilot testing of those guidelines; the agency released two guidelines in March 1992, intending to make several more available that summer.[46] If such guidelines were to be widely used to audit physician choices, the degree of bureaucratization in medical care would increase substantially. The requirement that physicians "clear" a large proportion of their decisions could impose significant additional costs in a system where, experts estimate, as much as 20 percent of expenditures already go to administrative matters,[47] and where provider frustration with the micromanagement of care is already intense.[48] Still, the movement has generated tremendous enthusiasm and significant funding. It is worth exploring the probable consequences of extending its approach to other types of "wasteful" care.

Treatment of Uncertain Effectiveness

Dr. Ellwood's estimate that "half of what the medical profession does is of unverified effectiveness"[49] is undeniably provocative. If that were the case, policymakers might well be advised to discontinue such practices pending scientific demonstration of their worth. Although this could mean waiting decades for research results, the successful implementation of this policy might cut medical costs dramatically.[50]

There is ample room for doubt about the effectiveness of many medical treatments. For some treatments, there are very few data on effectiveness. For most treatments, there is disagreement as to how to interpret the available data. In the face of this uncertainty, how feasible is it to talk about cutting waste with rules prohibiting payment for treatments of unverified effectiveness?

Most physicians would almost certainly oppose this approach. Because of the lack of scientific knowledge about disease, the practice of medicine is not a cookbook endeavor. Clinicians extrapolate beyond scientific data in "the large portion of cases . . . [that] are clinically gray and require clinical judgment."[51] Judging how to proceed in questionable cases is part of what constitutes the art of medicine. Physician Donald Berwick of the Harvard Community Health Plan has rightly warned that in choosing to cut waste by overriding clinical judgment, "we [may] gain control of care patterns only to find that care is being given by doctors who have lost pride and heart."[52] And while the specter of disheartened physicians might not forestall officials intent upon cutting costs, public opinion would likely inhibit this approach to cutting waste. Some patients would surely be outraged at being denied treatment simply because scientific data are lacking. The relatively minor turbulence that has attended the denial of "questionable" drugs to AIDS patients, along with the success that AIDS advocates have had in modifying and bypassing bureaucratic obstacles, foreshadows the uproar that would attend widespread denial of "questionable" care. For example, the constituency of patients with heart disease is unquestionably broader and more powerful than those with AIDS; many of the well-established technologies in this area are of uncertain benefit for many types of patients. It is implausible to expect that heart-disease victims would quietly forgo potentially lifesaving treatment in the name of scientific purity. In short, if "wasteful" means "of unverified effectiveness," cutting waste by making rules faces substantial popular and professional opposition.

Treatment That Is Ethically Troubling

The explosive growth of the bioethics field, an area that was virtually nonexistent a generation ago, testifies to the proliferation of ethically troubling medical treatment.[53] The use of aggressive medical therapies in treating the very old, the very young, and the very sick has engendered some of the most vehement charges of waste, inappropriateness, and irrationality in American medicine.

Rulemaking in this area requires an ethical consensus concerning an appropriate level of care. For people who are intimately acquainted with instances of gross overtreatment, this often seems a trivial problem. Waste is apparent and outrageous. Something like Justice Stewart's standard for obscenity—"I know it when I see it"—seems to hold. But experience shows that even the seemingly clearest cases can evoke controversy (if not litigation), bringing into conflict those most intimately familiar with the patient's situation. These controversies often reflect fundamental disagreements about the goals and obligations of providers, payers, and patients, or even disputes about the significance of human life, including a "right to life." We will not recapitulate the bioethical debates surrounding these issues.[54] It is enough to note that the term "wasteful" is used here in an entirely different sense than in the previous two sections. No literature search or scientific experiment satisfactorily speaks to this issue of waste. No consensus panel can settle the ethical question of what is futile, desirable, or even cruel.

What then are the possibilities for policy in this area? What kinds of rules can be made to cut waste in ethically problematic cases? Significant progress has been made in defining when it is *permissible* to terminate care. Guidelines developed in the bioethics community have informed court decisions and state statutes.[55] Such policies undoubtedly can help in guiding individual decisions, but their impact on the overall allocation of medical resources is unknown. Such guidelines, however, are not analogous to the RAND/Value procedures to cut waste. Little progress has been made in developing analogous rules in this area, rules that would say when wastefulness makes it *obligatory* to deny or terminate care. (It should be emphasized, moreover, that no one connected with the landmark RAND studies has proposed that any such rules be made.)

Their very suggestion is enormously controversial, as illustrated by the reception that greeted Daniel Callahan's proposal that age be a criterion in the allocation of public funds for medical care.[56] Highlighted on the op-ed pages of the *New York Times*,[57] the proposal drew vociferous attacks from gerontologists, senior-citizen advocates, and the elderly themselves. Social critic Nat Hentoff branded the scheme "morally depraved," a comment that was duly noted in the American Association of Retired People's *News Bulletin*.[58] Further discussion was effectively ended. If "wasteful" means "ethically troubling," cutting

wasteful care means facing hard and bitter choices. In matters of life
and death, when values clash, proposing allocational rules can place
those rules beyond reasonable public discussion. It is difficult to imagine
how such a process could lead to public consensus.

Treatment That Is Not Allocationally Efficient

Notwithstanding the above difficulties, bread-and-butter medicine is not about complex ethical issues. Rather, increasingly it is about
expensive medical care options. Today's physicians must choose daily
from among various costly treatments and tests, many of which are
unquestionably beneficial. Consider these lifesaving treatments:

(1) *Early cancer detection* (e.g., annual mammography for women
aged 40–50). Since women in this age group have a low incidence of
breast cancer, annual mammography offers a modest improvement in
life expectancy at a significant financial and social cost. Screening 25
percent of all American women in this age group on an annual basis
would save 373 lives each year. Costs (in 1984 dollars) would be $408
million for mammography, surgical workups, and continuing care. Savings from early detection of cancer would be $6 million annually, re-
sulting in a net annual cost of $402 million dollars to save 373 lives.[59]

(2) *Safer diagnostic tests* (e.g., nonionic contrast medium). Contrast
medium is a liquid which, when injected into the bloodstream, circulates
throughout the body making blood vessels and certain organs more
visible on x-ray. Injection with a dye carries a certain risk of a fatal
allergic reaction. Recently, a nonionic contrast dye was introduced that
is safer for patients. The risk of death from injection with the new dye
is 1 in 250,000 (an improvement over the risk of 1 in 30,000 with the
older dye). The newer dye costs ten times as much as the older one,
and widespread adoption could cost as much as $1 billion annually
nationwide.[60]

(3) *Organ transplantation* (e.g., heart transplantation). Heart replacement is surprisingly effective in the treatment of end-stage heart disease.
Recipients enjoy a 75–80 percent one-year survival rate. Although only
346 cardiac transplants were performed in 1984, an estimated 50,000
people could benefit from the procedure each year. Heart transplantation costs between $70,000 and $200,000 per patient.[61]

When do expensive maneuvers become "wasteful"? Traditionally,
policymakers have approached this problem from the framework of
cost-benefit analysis.[62] Given a rank ordering of medical programs and

procedures, beginning with the one with the best cost-to-benefit profile and ending with the one with the least attractive profile, one might simply allocate money from the top down. Above some cutoff point, the listed interventions could be considered worthwhile; below that point, wasteful. There are, however, three significant obstacles to implementing such a plan in American medicine.

The first is the nonavailability of a defensible rank ordering. We have scant information about the effectiveness and costs of most clinical interventions. Moreover, we lack a firm conceptual and empirical basis for equating different kinds of medical, social, and financial benefits. In the absence of these two sorts of information, it is difficult to assign meaningful cost-benefit estimates to medical procedures.[63] The second difficulty is that the American medical care system does not operate within a fixed budget (nor do most American physicians). Without a budgetary limit, the borderline between worthwhile and wasteful simply cannot be defined. It is impossible to say which interventions would fall below a purely hypothetical cutoff. A final obstacle arises from our decentralized system of financing. We have no guarantee that cuts in wasteful expenditures will be compensated with shifts toward worthwhile expenditures. We may agree that annual mammographic screening for young women is comparatively wasteful, but we have no reason to believe that money saved by abstaining from mammography will be spent on a more worthwhile endeavor, such as universal access to prenatal care.

While rigorous cost-benefit analysis is unlikely to govern the allocation of medical services in the foreseeable future, concerns about costs and benefits will continue to have an important place in discussions of wasteful care. This is surely appropriate, since no medical care system can provide all possible services. But when "not cost-effective" is taken to be synonymous with "wasteful," some misleading inferences can follow. One of these is the suggestion that treatments that fall below the cost-benefit cutoff point are wasteful and therefore do no one much good. This is certainly not true. There are many potentially lifesaving treatments that are very costly, but effective (breast-cancer screening in young women, safer diagnostic tests, and organ transplantation all fall into this category). When cutting waste on economic grounds, we inevitably eliminate some services that do some good. We should therefore not be surprised to find people fighting for access to treatments that are "not cost-effective," as did the members of the Komen Foundation for Breast Cancer in Dallas, a group of wealthy and socially prominent Republican women who successfully lobbied the Texas legislature in 1989 to require that insurance companies cover the cost of screening mammography for all women ages 35 and over.[64]

Such episodes lay bare the link between waste cutting and rationing. If "waste cutting" means "trimming the fat," and "rationing" means "making rules to limit the use of beneficial services," it will necessarily be the case that in trimming fat we deny some people some beneficial services. What is particularly striking is that the *perception* of benefit determines the political cost of waste cutting. While the medical costs of denying young women access to screening mammography are quite small (as the analysis cited above demonstrates), the political price may be prohibitive (as the Texas legislators found out). Similarly, in the recent Oregon rationing movement, procedures were initially ranked according to their alleged cost-to-benefit profiles. Organ transplants were near the bottom in this initial list of services, but the political costs of cutting this form of so-called waste were seen as too great, and organ transplants were moved upward on the list so that they would qualify for Medicare reimbursement.[65] Cutting waste, when waste is either of great benefit or is perceived to be so, can be prohibitively expensive politically.

More generally, economically driven rulemaking runs counter to those American values and institutions favoring aggressive, high-technology, "do something" medicine. Opinion polls show that Americans believe, nearly unanimously, that financial considerations should not enter into life-and-death medical decisions.[66] In the legal arena, technological imperatives dovetail with our shared notions of individual rights and professional responsibilities, meaning that rulemaking could exacerbate an increasingly unacceptable malpractice environment. As people who are injured by denial of care seek restitution, several issues will be at stake: Can care be denied because it is too expensive? When harm results from denial of treatment, who is responsible? What are the responsibilities of payers and providers? Already, some interesting cases have been heard. A Washington state court recently held that a third-party payer had a duty to pay for a man's liver transplant because his life depended on it.[67] A Michigan woman with colon cancer has sued her HMO, maintaining that its cost-containment rules led to a delay in the detection of her malignancy.[68]

While commentators agree that the relationship between the malpractice standard and care cost containment is one of the most important issues confronting medical tort law in the 1990s, they are divided on how the legal system will accommodate rulemaking. Some argue that physicians who prudently adopt recommended sparer practice styles will find protection in the event of adverse outcomes.[69] Others are doubtful that the accommodation can be made so smoothly, and fear that economically based rulemaking will "create enormous confusion and, quite likely, place physicians under inappropriate and unfair economic and legal pressures"[70] as they are forced to make choices between their own professional standards and payers' rules.

Whatever the political and legal outcomes, it is clear that economically driven rulemaking could force physicians to redefine their professional roles. Many physicians find such rulemaking unacceptable,[71] and many believe that cost-containment measures seriously compromise the quality of medical care.[72] Some hold that consideration of costs simply has no place in the practice of medicine. One frequently quoted passage draws a parallel between the obligations of physicians to their patients and the responsibilities of attorneys to their clients:

> Physicians are required to do everything that they believe may benefit each patient without regard to costs or other societal considerations. In caring for an individual patient, the doctor must act solely as that patient's advocate, against the apparent interests of society as a whole, if necessary. An analogy can be drawn with the role of a lawyer defending a client against a criminal charge. The attorney is obligated to use all ethical means to defend the client, regardless of the cost of prolonged legal proceedings or even of the possibility that a guilty person may be acquitted through skillful advocacy. Similarly, in the practice of medicine, physicians are obligated to do all that they can for their patients without regard to any costs to society.[73]

This attitude, which one might call the "professional imperative," dominates American medical practice, and it will not disappear overnight.

REALISTIC PROSPECTS FOR RULEMAKING

This brief survey of the policy to cut waste by rulemaking has revealed that it is really many policies—at least as many policies as there are kinds of waste. Three summary points should be emphasized. First, there are different senses in which treatments are "wasteful." We know that some treatments are wasteful by looking at their results; in other cases we need to examine their price tag; in still others we must make a moral judgment. While this is not a profound point, it is one that is frequently obscured in the rhetoric of waste cutting. Medicare's rules about medical necessity (and myriad similarly disingenuous policies) create confusion, breed cynicism, and offer little promise as long-term strategies to guide the allocation of medical service.[74]

Second, since waste is diverse, policies to cut waste face different prospects for success. Although some forms of care can probably be prohibited with little resistance, this is not likely to be the case generally. There will be substantial professional, political, ethical, and legal obstacles to cutting waste in many cases. Although identification of wasteful practices may be conceptually straightforward, the costs of rule-making may be high. Rules can work, but these obstacles must be faced squarely in attempts to develop coherent and realistic health policy.

Third, because the spectrum of "wasteful" care includes care that is effective, cutting waste by making rules will not always circumvent hard choices. Sometimes it may mean eliminating care that is both needed and beneficial. In other cases, it may mean cutting services that are perceived to be beneficial but are of uncertain effectiveness. In either case, we must watch out for immoderate promises about painless waste cutting.

While doubts about rulemaking are warranted, nihilism is not. We all stand to gain from the knowledge that will flow from the outcomes movement, and rulemaking may work in some situations. As we have shown, *rulemaking is likely to be particularly successful when the treatment in question is clearly ineffective or harmful*. It is, however, far from obvious that such instances are sufficiently prevalent to justify the extravagant optimism surrounding the movement's likely impact. While the oft-cited RAND study of three commonly performed procedures showed that they were performed "inappropriately" in one-third to one-sixth of the cases,[75] this figure in all likelihood overstates the prevalence of ineffective or harmful care for three reasons. First, the three procedures were apparently chosen precisely because the indications for their use are unclear. Given this uncertainty, it is not surprising that they were often used "inappropriately." Second, the RAND ratings were based on a retrospective review of medical records. It is likely that incomplete documentation produced a number of cases incorrectly rated as inappropriate.[76] This interpretation is supported by data from two published cases in which the appropriateness criteria were used prospectively. In both cases, inappropriateness rates were simply not as impressive as might have been hoped. In the early Aetna/Value trial, only 9 percent of the proposed services were ultimately deemed not appropriate for reimbursement.[77] In a more recent trial of the Value software at five Blue Cross and Blue Shield plans, preauthorization review yielded a judgment of inappropriateness for 11 percent of the cases overall.[78]

Let us assume that 11 percent of all present medical practices are demonstrably ineffective or harmful. Eliminating those wasteful practices would result in substantial savings, given our present level of expenditure—an attractive prospect indeed. But are savings of that magnitude likely to be realized in the near future? It seems likely that implementation would take place over a period of years, given the AHCPR's past (and admirable) record of crafting guidelines carefully.[79] After developing guidelines, a strategy will have to be developed to change physician behavior. Whether that strategy relies on "education"—as the AHCPR would apparently prefer[80]—or on a RAND/Value-like direct linkage to reimbursement,[81] it is clear that it would begin to have its intended effect only after a period of years.

If this is the case, how can rulemaking affect our level of medical care spending over the next decade? Providing a precise answer to this question would require us to address issues of health economics that are beyond the scope of the present chapter. But one can see that the possible 11 percent savings—particularly a savings achieved gradually—would inevitably be dwarfed by the losses exacted by the present rate of medical care inflation, which one expert has estimated to occur at a real rate of 7 percent per annum.[82] Unfortunately, the plan to cut waste by making rules simply does not address this cost, one of the central problems of health services allocation. Eliminating today's waste cannot help us constrain the escalation of costs attributable to the more effective and more expensive services to be developed tomorrow. Viewed from this perspective, cutting waste by making rules is, at best, an incremental reform that might produce modest gains over the medium term. Despite the claims of its more ardent supporters, it shows little promise as a solution to the so-called health care cost crisis.

In the end, the parameters movement may founder—not because of a lack of "wasteful" medical care, but because government and business leaders want a quicker fix to the problem of rising medical care costs. With wasteful care on the public's mind, a coalition of resourceful researchers, government officials, politicians, business leaders, and professional organizations have developed a vision of a world in which scientific know-how aided by computerized wizardry will produce rules for allocating the "right" amount of medical care. But the public's issue-attention cycle waxes and wanes quickly.[83] As it becomes clear that it would be years before hoped-for economic gains could be realized, and that cuts in waste entail significant social costs, the movement could lose some of its momentum and funding. As the AHCPR's director remarked to an audience of health-services researchers:

> We have a wonderful opportunity to make outcomes and effectiveness research a very important incremental chapter in the pursuit of quality and value for the health care dollar. I believe that window is only going to be open so long. The Congress indeed expects things tomorrow, and I believe that with reasonable progress reports from you, I can be a part of telling them that good work takes time. At the same time, if we say that it takes five to six years and please hold your breath, then I think we'll lose. So as I said to the [outcomes research] teams that were assembled here a few days ago, we're delighted at the progress you're making, but hurry up.[84]

IS THERE AN ALTERNATIVE TO RULEMAKING?

Nothing above is intended to imply that there is a simple solution to the problem of rising medical expenditures. The professional imperative that drives physicians to provide more, better, and safer services (and the desire for better health that drives patients to seek the same) will continue. If we are to curb rising costs, powerful countervailing forces must be brought to bear. Rules can certainly help in applying such forces, and the parameters movement is well under way. But is rulemaking the most promising course of action? Any answer must take into account two decades of frustrating failure to contain health expenditures in America. During that time, there were numerous attempts to change the way in which America delivers, pays for, and regulates medical care. None has been demonstrably successful in curbing medical care inflation or in constraining the growth in the intensity of services provided. Neither competition, managed care, prospective payment, nor numerous other purported panaceas has fulfilled its promise. Each in its day was touted as the answer to the problem of rising costs, leading to cycles of delight and disappointment as expenditures resumed their seemingly inexorable rise, or costs were shifted onto other sectors of the medical care economy.[85] To expect more of the outcomes movement would be to ignore the lessons of experience. It is worth sketching what these lessons might be.

During the same 20-year period that costs rose in this country, other nations had substantially greater success in controlling health expenditures. Canada's and Britain's systems are most often cited, but most of Western Europe's achievements are comparable.[86] In each case, the inherently inflationary forces in medical care that Robert Evans has so eloquently described—technological growth, asymmetry of information, uncertainty of evidence, and rising expectations—have been met with policy responses to counter powerful pressures for more spending. In Canada, that has meant the concentration of financial authority in single provincial payers, the use of global hospital budgets, the separate control of capital expenditures by hospitals, and the active setting of prices for physician services. In the United States, reforms failed to address those forces in a concerted fashion, and inflation continued unabated.[87]

There are indications that America is moving toward universal health insurance. Public opinion polls show that a majority of Americans favor a national health insurance system over our present arrangements.[88] The appearance in the elite *New England Journal of Medicine* of an editorial[89] and an article[90] supporting some form of universal health insurance signaled that the academic wing of the medical profession is ready to consider fundamental changes in the way that medical care is financed. An entire issue of the *Journal of the American Medical Association* extolled the virtues of universal access,[91] suggesting that others will not be far behind. The Congress appears prepared to consider such a program seriously for the first time in 25 years.[92]

Still, most of these powerful parties are unconvinced that reform should include the kind of concentrated financial and regulatory power that has repeatedly proved successful abroad. In the context of the federal budget deficit and the public's hostility toward increased taxes, it is uncertain whether reform will follow the model of direct governmental financing. Some claim that a system that preserves the present employment-based insurance scheme and maintains some role for private insurance companies is politically more feasible.[93] If such a program could be coupled with strong governmental regulatory powers, some observers believe that we might achieve universal access to medical care, while still containing costs.[94]

As the debate on major reforms heightens over the coming months, one truth will continue to be undeniable: contemporary medicine offers an astonishing array of beneficial therapies. These therapies will be sought by many patients wanting to improve their lives. They will be employed by doctors wanting to help their patients, exercise their craft, and carn their income. There is little hope that either of the intimate partners in the doctor-patient relationship will come to see most medical treatment as wasteful.

Meanwhile, the professional imperative will prevail unless powerfully constrained. While many physicians will refrain from performing procedures known to be ineffective, most will not be willing to unilaterally cut other "wasteful" activities (practices of uncertain effectiveness, activities that are ethically problematic, and therapies that are not allocationally efficient). If doctors will not say no to their patients, then we can expect that payers will begin to say no to doctors. And indeed they have begun to do so. A new coalition has promised to cut health expenditures by making rules forbidding wasteful treatment. But it is doubtful that cutting waste is as straightforward or as painless as the most voluble members of the coalition have suggested. And it is certain that cutting waste by making rules will mean different things to different people.

Chapter 6
Rationing: Painful Prescription,
Inadequate Diagnosis

WITH RUDOLF KLEIN

American medicine is in trouble. Its costs are staggering. Its record of performance—on access, effectiveness, and efficiency—is mixed. And its future worries millions of Americans.

The United States is a laggard among its Organization for Economic Cooperation and Development (OECD) counterparts in health status. In life expectancy, American males rank fifteenth and American females seventh in the world. More than a dozen countries have lower infant mortality rates and, comparatively, Americans are losing ground.[1]

These shortcomings contrast starkly with accomplishments of which

From "Cost vs. Care: America's Health Care Dilemma Wrongly Considered," *Health Matrix*, Vol. 4, No. 1 (Spring 1986), pp. 19–24. Reprinted by permission.

This essay is adapted, with considerable revision, from a lecture delivered at Brown University on March 13, 1985. The opening section is partly drawn from T. R. Marmor and A. Dunham, "The Politics of Health Policy Reform: Problems, Origins, Alternatives, and a Possible Prescription" in *Health Care: How to Improve It and Pay for It* (Washington, D.C.: Center for National Policy, 1985). The section on the use of British evidence in American health policy debate is taken from the unpublished article by Rudolf Klein and Theodore Marmor, "Painful Prescription: The Inadequate Diagnosis." Professor Marmor's work has been generously supported by the Henry J. Kaiser Family Foundation, Menlo Park, California.

107

Table 6.1
National health expenditures

Calendar year	Total amount (in billions)	Percent of GNP
1960	$ 26.9	5.3
1970	74.7	7.5
1980	249.0	9.5
1981	286.6	9.8
1982	322.4	10.5
1983	355.4	10.8
Projections 1984	392.7	10.9
1987	529.8	11.6
1990	690.4	12.3

Source: Mark S. Freeland and Carol E. Schendler, "Health Spending in the 1980s," *Health Care Financing Review,* Vol. 5, No. 3 (Spring 1984): 7.

American medicine can be justifiably proud. Among these we can count sharp increases in life expectancy in the last two and a half decades, preventive vaccines for many often fatal diseases and cures for still others, and remarkable new diagnostic tools and life-prolonging technology.

The United States is not, however, a laggard when it comes to medical spending. Medical costs have soared for two and a half decades. The country spent $322 billion for medical care in 1982, 10.5 percent of Gross National Product (GNP).[2] In 1983, a year when the general inflation rate was only 3.9 percent, this figure increased 10.3 percent to $355.4 billion, or 10.8 percent of GNP.[3] Under present policies, the nation's medical care bill was projected to reach some $700 billion in 1990, 12.3 percent of GNP (See Table 6.1).[4] Rising costs affect everyone: individuals, as out-of-pocket costs and health insurance premiums rise at alarming rates; employers, who pay more than 80 percent of the cost of health insurance premiums; government at all levels, as Medicare, Medicaid, and local government expenditures continue to increase rapidly; and the nation, as medical care appropriates an ever-increasing share of our resources.

America spends over $2 billion per day on medical care, but too much of it is misspent. Properly expended, there are more than enough financial resources to pay for decent care for every American. As it is, however, American medical care is neither equitable nor efficient.

Millions of Americans do not receive the care they need while money is squandered on unneeded, unwanted, and sometimes even harmful services and unnecessary facilities. An estimated 40 percent of minority women receive no prenatal care during the first trimester of pregnancy. One-fifth of the nation's children are not immunized against polio and only half our children are fully immunized against preventable childhood diseases.[5] Almost 900 counties have fewer than one doctor per 3,500 people, leaving thousands of communities without basic care.[6] American workers find their employers forced either to cut back on their health benefits or to restrict wages to pay for increasing medical costs. Health insurance for ordinary Americans is eroding, leaving too many unprotected or underprotected. For the first time in 30 years, from 1979 to 1982 the number of Americans without health insurance increased.[7] In 1983, 14 percent—one out of every seven Americans—reported that they could not get the care they needed because of cost, many because of unemployment.[8] Financial barriers to access, let alone equal access, grew much higher in the 1980s, leaving some 30 million Americans underserved.

At the same time, we waste money on inefficient and often ineffective services and facilities. Physicians order whole batteries of tests of doubtful utility but do not take time to talk with or examine patients. Many hospital beds are filled unnecessarily with patients who could be treated as outpatients, or treated elsewhere, or who do not need treatment at all. Increased use of life-prolonging technology has led to a situation in which medicine too often prolongs dying, not living.

Medical inflation—particularly for hospital care—remains one-and-one-half to two times the rate of general price increases. That inflation, despite recent decreases from the hyper-rates of 1982–1983, continues to put severe financial strains on families, on American business, and on government budgets. State health spending has been rising much faster than the willingness of many states to pay for it. And spending for health constitutes a significant part of current and projected federal budget deficits.

The United States faces the challenge of making access to affordable care a reality rather than an empty promise. In 1965, the passage of Medicare and Medicaid symbolized that promise to the elderly and the poor. Today we face the continued erosion of that promise. But no one is interested in cost containment as an end in itself. If medical inflation can be controlled sensibly, the United States can turn its attention to improving our uneven patchwork of public and private health insurance and promoting our health in other ways.

Must we, in addressing that task, confront a cruel dilemma of cost versus care? Must Americans, as Dr. William Schwartz claimed in *Newsweek* in the fall of 1984, "either . . . accept the high and rising cost of hospital care or . . . eventually have to ration it?"[9] Great Britain, he went on to say, "has long since taken the course and made its peace with it." According to Schwartz, we are on the horns of a dilemma: either pay more for health care or cut off some lifesaving technology, the very sort of thing people worry about when they are sick. This view, to my mind, presents a false dichotomy. It muddies the discussion about cost containment in the United States and contributes to illusions about our choices by questionable inferences from British medical and financial experience. That is the sense in which the cost versus care dilemma is "wrongly considered."

THE USE OF BRITISH EVIDENCE IN AMERICAN HEALTH POLICY DEBATES

A specter stalks the perennial American debate on cost containment. It is the specter of Britain's National Health Service (NHS). If the United States were to clamp down on the growth of spending, if it were to impose a strict global budget on the British model, then inevitably it would have to follow the example of the NHS and ration health care. Instead of being available on demand, health care would be allocated by physicians according to their own criteria of need and priorities. The result, it is argued, would be to import into the United States the British system of queuing and waiting lists. The case, as it is usually presented, is designed to evoke horror and revulsion and to persuade the audience that anything remotely resembling the British system would be unacceptable in the United States.

The 1984 book by Aaron and Schwartz—combining the perspectives of an economist and a physician—attempts to disentangle facts from myth. In *The Painful Prescription: Rationing Hospital Care,* Aaron and Schwartz address the question of just how Britain's NHS rations health care by examining how its provision of certain therapeutic procedures compares with the provision in the United States.[10] The result is a methodologically rigorous descriptive study that threatens to create a new myth because of the assumptions underlying its analysis, and the conclusions unwary readers might draw on the basis of the presented interpretations.

Aaron and Schwartz are, of course, not responsible for the misinterpretations of others. But they have contributed to the mischief in three ways. First, their investigation of British medical politics is characteristically marred by overly simple generalizations. For example, *Painful Prescription* makes the unusual contention that "to an American, the most striking aspect of the creation of the National Health Service in 1948 was the relative lack of controversy over the event."[11] Citing as authority the British Information Services guide on the subject, Aaron and Schwartz largely ignore the scholarship by political scientists, sociologists, and historians on the origins of the highly complex NHS,[12] a story of considerable party agreement on principle and ferocious dispute on particulars.

Superficial on the texture of British politics, Aaron and Schwartz are largely silent on the logic of cross-national policy studies. While exceedingly useful as portraits of medical practice in two societies, *Painful Prescription,* as its very title indicates, is a book primarily directed at influencing American public policy. And despite their expressed caution, the authors are hardly cautious. In their *New England Journal of Medicine* article, they boldly claim to have found "lessons from Britain." Despite the differences, "the British experiment," they say, "has yielded the best data we are likely to find in advance of embarking on an intensive program to curb medical expenditures."[13] The foreword to their book, taking its cue from the authors' emphasis rather than their occasional caveats, cites *Painful Prescription*'s "use of the British experiences as the basis for drawing inferences about how Americans would respond should they undertake to sharply reduce growth of medical spending."[14]

Third, the authors have drawn inferences from British experience that are not supported by the more relevant Canadian evidence on cost control and rationing. Because they ignored the Canadian experience, their claim that there is a sharp dichotomy between rising costs and severe rationing in the not-to-distant future appears less implausible. Had we in the United States just matched Canada's experience in the 1970s, our outlays would have been roughly one-fifth less than our current spending. That means some $70 billion less in 1983 dollars, hardly a minor matter on the way to eventual severe rationing. And

Canada accomplished its cost control without anything close to the levels of service rationing of Britain.[15]

The main findings of the Aaron and Schwartz study can be summarized quickly. Some therapeutic procedures are as readily available in Britain as in the United States: treatment of hemophilia, bone marrow transplantation, and megavoltage radiotherapy. Others, however, "are clearly rationed when compared with the United States." The overall rate of treatment for chronic renal failure in Britain is less than half that in the United States; the rate of coronary artery surgery in Britain is only 10 percent of that of the United States; the British hospital system has only one-fifth to one-tenth as many intensive-care beds as the United States relative to population; Britain has only one-sixth the computerized tomography (CT) scanning capacity of the United States.

The problems start with the interpretation of these findings and, despite Aaron and Schwartz's intermittent efforts to be cautious, the uses to which their interpretations will be put in American health debates. Throughout their study, Aaron and Schwartz use rates of provision and use in the United States as their initial benchmark for assessing the performance of the NHS. They explain that, except for cases where they have evidence of overprovision in the United States, they "regard Britain as providing full care if it provides care as frequently and in the same general way as the United States does."[16] Given the evidence of overprovision and overuse in the United States—particularly of various surgical and diagnostic procedures—it is far from self-evident that the American model provides the best starting point for assessing the performance of other health care systems, or its own.

Why, one might well ask, would scholars of American medical care policy and politics turn to Britain's experience at all? Surely, as Aaron and Schwartz rightly note, the cultural and economic wealth differences are too great to conceive of wholesale importation of particular British health policies. Britain, after all, is a relatively poor industrial nation, with a unified parliamentary regime, a class structure far more rigid than that of the United States, and a spectrum of political ideologies far wider than America's.

For purposes of estimating what American politics might do with an imported policy—like the British form of powerful central budgeting and clinical autonomy—the right method is to explore national circumstances and experiences as similar as possible to America's. Were direct simulation their purpose, estimating what centralized budgeting caps would work like in American, Canadian, Australian, and German experience would have been a more promising subject than British rationing. Aaron and Schwartz, attentive to the methodology of medical description, are silent on the logic of comparative policy studies.

COMPARATIVE METHODS

Broadly speaking, there are two quite different reasons for comparing social policies across nations, each of which would seem to require a rather different research strategy. First, there is what we call *policy learning*.[17] That is, we look at the social policies of other countries in order to derive lessons or models which can be applied at home. This approach has a long history. Presidential commissions and European royal commissions regularly draw on the experience of other countries: see, for instance, the American Report of the Committee on Economic Security in 1935.[18]

Second, there is what we call *policy understanding*. Here the emphasis is not so much on learning as on explanation. For example, if we are to achieve an understanding of the factors which shape the evolution of a social security system, it is unlikely that we can do so by looking at one country in isolation. Are the key variables the level of industrialization and the political mobilization of the working class? The history of Britain, examined in isolation, might suggest that they are. But comparative studies indicate otherwise.[19] Similarly, it has been argued that in Britain the power of the medical profession rests on its access to Whitehall,[20] while comparative studies show that the nature of that power is largely independent of the precise relationship between doctors and bureaucracy.[21] In short, comparative studies may be essential if misleading conclusions are not to be drawn from what are single-case studies in the creation or evolution of social policy.

The research strategy associated with the first of these two approaches would, to judge from the literature, seem to be a micro strategy (or single-issue approach) in "most similar" countries, keeping numbers down. That is, the prime concern is not with the nature of the social policy *system,* since it is implausible to assume that a total system can be transplanted from one country to another, but with a discrete area of policy. In turn, this means comparing countries that are judged to be roughly similar in terms of economic development, social organization, and political ideology. For if the focus of concern is the transplantability of ideas or models, then it is clearly essential that the two environments not be too different.

The research strategy associated with the second approach would seem to be a macro strategy (or systems approach) in "most different" countries, using large numbers. In this approach, the focus of interest is on the factors that help to explain either the evolution or the behavior of the system as a whole. The nature of the analysis positively requires differences in the economic development, social organization, or political ideology of the countries being examined (for it is impossible to test the significance of a specific factor if it is common to all the cases being examined). Large numbers, insofar as they allow a statistical analysis of the factors concerned, are an additional advantage.

Aaron and Schwartz have applied a variant of the "different system" approach to Britain's experience. Such analyses address an admittedly very different sociopolitical community, contrast its practices with another country, and highlight the cultural and other factors which set the two societies apart. Given profound cultural differences, one sees them more clearly by asking similar questions of the two cultures.

Anthropologists do this for a living, but the practice has its own tradition of caution in drawing any policy lessons at all. The legitimate purpose of this variant is analytical illumination without policy transplantation.

In employing this approach, Aaron and Schwartz explicitly make the caveats about how different the American experience would be with British models. "Within the British hospital, [the overall budget limit] decision is made on a collegial basis by consultants, subject to peer pressure, and by district and regional planning officials, not all of whom are doctors," but, they acknowledge, "the situation in the United States is quite different."[22] And the differences they are careful to identify would mean that, for the United States, "the stresses [of severe budgetary limits] at first would be much less severe and the decisions less draconian," but that "the restrictions would be perceived as more painful."[23]

But they take away with one hand what they give with the other. At one point, Aaron and Schwartz cautiously assert that their readers "will have to decide whether we tell a plausible story about why the British have the limited care they have and whether people in the United States would respond similarly or differently."[24] And they remind us that the "important differences between British and American society and medical practice . . . prevent us from using British experience as an exact script for the choices the United States would make if it sought to curb medical expenditures."[25] They state that they themselves "are persuaded that the United States is not interested in creating a national health service on the British model" and must therefore "rely on other means."[26] On the other hand, however, we are told that the differences "do not invalidate the relevance of these experiences and choices for the United States."[27] One cannot in logic be green and white all over at the same time. And, in cross-national policy studies, one cannot say that another national experience is both profoundly different and a useful guide to a very dissimilar society.

The appropriate approach to British experience, then, is one of understanding differences in medical systems, of illuminating how those different medical systems work, and of explaining their character. The real challenge, when trying to compare the American and British health care systems, is to try to disentangle the reasons for differences in the rate of provision and use.

INTERPRETATIONS

Differences obviously reflect a variety of factors. They may reflect differences in the availability of resources, the most obvious explanation when comparing a country that spends only 6 percent of its GNP with one that spends over 10 percent. They may reflect differences in the incentives to physicians: the United States fee-for-service system clearly gives doctors an incentive to maximize activity, while the British system of salaried hospital doctors provides an incentive to minimize activity (to caricature only a little). Finally, they may reflect different traditions of clinical practice and different views about what good medical practice actually involves.

The trouble, of course, is that all these factors are linked. In the case of the United States, the open-ended nature of the financial commitment to health care means that physicians can maximize their own incomes by adopting, as Aaron and Schwartz recognize, an aggressive approach to medical treatment. The environment allows the professional imperative to be defined in terms of throwing everything possible—considering technology and resources—at the patient, irrespective of the chances of actually "curing" him or her. In the case of Britain, the result of the system of global budgets set for each hospital is that physicians are acutely aware that one patient who is overtreated means in terms of the available resources that another patient may be undertreated, or not be treated at all. The environment nudges physicians to adopt a conservative, cautious approach to treatment and forces them to be selective in their use of medical technology in its widest sense—as in the use of diagnostic procedures.

One conclusion drawn by Aaron and Schwartz is that in Britain this situation persuades physicians to disguise rationing decisions as clinical decisions. Physicians internalize, as it were, the resource constraints and lower their clinical sights accordingly. To an extent this is true. Renal dialysis is a good example of resource constraints, where undoubtedly some patients are turned away to die on ostensibly clinical criteria (although it is not at all clear what the quality of their lives would be if extended; on this point, the study offers only modest assurance). But in other cases the conclusion does not follow on the basis of the evidence offered. Cautious use of diagnostic procedures or chemotherapy for cancer may simply reflect a humane concern for the patient and an unwillingness to subject him or her to procedures which are unlikely to yield either significantly greater diagnostic certainty or life expectancy. More important still, Aaron and Schwartz fail to emphasize the reverse conclusion for the United States—that an abundance of resources may persuade physicians to internalize their own desire to experiment with new techniques or to increase their incomes and transmute their own personal preferences into heroic medical practices. Given this central flaw in their analysis, their statistics of comparative activity are easily misinterpreted.

This said, Aaron and Schwartz are undoubtedly right in their contention that the British NHS gives less priority than the United States system to "quality of life" treatments such as hip replacement. Although all the evidence suggests that the NHS copes fully and competently with life-threatening conditions, it does not adequately meet the demand for procedures designed to enhance the quality of life. Still, the length of queuing times in Britain is frequently exaggerated. For example, while there may be instances of people waiting years for a hip replacement operation, because they are classified as nonurgent cases, the median waiting time for orthopedic surgery is only 12 weeks. Aaron and Schwartz could have strengthened their case on this point by more extensive examination of the role of the private health care sector in Britain. Its expansion in recent years certainly provides evidence of unsatisfied demand for certain forms of relatively minor surgical procedures, such as for hernias and varicose veins.

All this is not to urge exporting Britain's NHS to the United States. The two systems are anchored in profound differences of professional culture between the two nations, which reflect the differences between the two societies. A system which works well in a paternalistic society like Britain, with its lingering if ebbing tradition of deference to professional experts, would not necessarily work in an entrepreneurial society like America, with its emphasis on the engineering of ever-higher expectations on the part of consumers. However, it is to argue that Britain's NHS should not be used as a specter to frighten off people from a system of health care based on global budgeting, a system which, if ever adopted in the United States, would no doubt have to be cast in a quite different mold to take account of very different circumstances. And it would be unfortunate indeed if the Aaron and Schwartz study were to be used to frighten Americans, despite its many merits.

The very specter of severe rationing confuses rather than clarifies the debate in the United States. There is no substantial support in the United States for the more ascetic style of British medicine. American patients, as Aaron and Schwartz themselves assert, would be strongly opposed to severe limits on lifesaving technology such as kidney dialysis. American politicians are not likely to press for draconian measures, except as scare tactics to ward off sensible cost control. As the Canadian example illustrates, it is possible to have American levels of medical care, in a comparably rich country, with considerable lower outlays. That means less income for those in medicine, a painful prescription indeed. But the political realities of conflict over constraining the incomes of the medical industry should not be confused with the specter of sharp reductions in the level of services provided.

CONCLUSION

Why do we regard the formulation of the cost versus care dilemma as misleading? Think about American medicine as we have described it, an industry that spends almost 11 percent of the GNP. It exists in a country where 25 to 30 million Americans are not covered for health insurance, a country in which close to 25 percent of Medicare's $60 million budget is spent for care in the last month of life.

Contrast that situation with the circumstances of our northern neighbor, Canada. Canada spends less than 10 percent of its GNP, roughly 2 percent less than we do, on health care. Canadian national health insurance provides comprehensive coverage for every Canadian man, woman, and child. In 1970, both nations were spending exactly the same proportion of GNP. Since 1970, Canada has stabilized the share of its national resources going to medical care while, during the same period, our share of national resources spent on medical care has grown from 7 percent to almost 11 percent.[28]

Let us add to this comparison. If you ask Canadians whether they are, on the whole, satisfied with the quality of care they get and with their access to the services that Canadian medicine provides, the overwhelming majority would say yes. Ask yourself also whether their society is more similar to ours than is Great Britain's, or to what extent the distribution of their population is similar to that of the United States. The truth is that Canada is, in almost every way, more comparable to the United States than to Great Britain. And if it is possible, in a society not identical but roughly comparable to ours, to provide comprehensive medical care at 2 percent less of GNP than we now spend, there would appear to be a very good basis for believing that we are spending more than necessary.

Let us look at the implications of this in quantitative terms. If 15 percent to 25 percent of what we now spend on medical care could be spent in other ways more effectively, or could be not spent at all, then it seems quite wrong to say that we are faced with the stark choice of either reducing the quantity of medical care or controlling its cost. In other words, there is a third way between the British example of severe service rationing in some areas and the American way of continued high spending on medical care. That third way is the Canadian route to cost containment—compatible with decent access to medical care.

The differences in expenditures in the two countries have been pointed out. The divergent patterns of the last 20 years that led to these differences need to be examined. During the period from 1950 to 1970, the experiences of the two countries—in terms of percentage of GNP spent on health and also in patterns of insurance expansion—were broadly identical. In the United States, we experienced expansion of public insurance, aimed at selected groups of the population; for example, Medicare for the elderly, Medicaid for the poor, to some extent expansion of veterans' coverage. Canada had public expansion by type of service: government insurance for hospital care in the late 1950s and for medical (physician) services in the late 1960s.

The first element in our comparison, then, is that Canada and the United States have had, in the postwar period, broadly similar experiences with medical care costs and with the expansion of insurance. Second, both societies can be understood as fragments of British political culture—the parliamentary model in Canada, and the presidential model in the United States.

Interestingly, while our political traditions in some ways are both grafted from a British base, we also experience another significant similarity—both America and Canada are largely immigrant societies. In the postwar period, both societies saw tremendous expansion of non-English-speaking groups. Chicago, for instance, is the second largest Polish city in the world, and Toronto has much the same degree of ethnic diversity. Close to a third of the Canadian provincial population comes from non-English-speaking backgrounds. So we find in both countries ethnic pluralism, British culture as the constitutional basis, and two societies with broadly comparable levels of economic wealth.

Most important, the medical care that is practiced, the medical education that is taught, and the type of hospitals that are operating are ones that both American and Canadian physicians recognize as broadly similar. They read the same journals, they have access to similar kinds of technology, and they experienced in the postwar period the same relentless growth of third-party financiers intervening in a world of professional autonomy.

These areas of similarity are the grounds for believing that, if the people in the United States were to try some of the cost-containment steps already taken in Canada, we have reason to believe that we could experience similar results. This is not to claim that we would have identical experiences. It is, however, to say that there are enough similarities between Canada and the United States to make an investigation of Canada's policy options relevant to our choices.

Let us conclude with a couple of considerations that ought to condition the way we think about the Canadian evidence. Almost thirty years ago, we made a promise to America's poor and America's old. We told them that, if they happened to be poor, other things might be a problem for them, but not medical care. Medicaid would bring them into the mainstream of American medicine. And we promised American senior citizens in the same year that, when they were old and sick, they would have access to American medical care in which their financial circumstances would not be the primary determinant of the care they received. Today these promises are eroding before our eyes. In the wake of the runaway medical inflation of the 1980s, and in the presence of the overpowering importance of the federal budget deficit, we are fixated on ways by which we can cut back government programs. In the case of Medicare, that means only three choices: costs will be shifted back on the elderly themselves, in which case their capacity to pay will, in part, determine their access to care; costs will be borne by other payers, like all of us, in third-party payments; or older people with less means will get different access to medical care than they used to have. Those are cruel choices, yet they are the real dilemmas of Medicare and medical care reform.

Part II

---

*The Debate over Universal
Health Insurance*

Chapter 7
American Medical Care Reform:
Are We Doomed to Fail?

WITH DAVID BOYUM

No one seriously doubts that American medical care needs reform. The most obvious problems are skyrocketing costs—in 1991, total health expenditures in the United States were an estimated $740 billion[1]—and the growing numbers of uninsured—more than 40 million Americans in any one year have no health insurance at all.[2] But the troubles only begin there.

Americans currently labor under a confusing and wasteful system of coverage. This haphazard mix includes privately purchased policies, government-provided insurance for the elderly (Medicare) and for some of the poor (Medicaid), Health Maintenance Organizations (HMOs) and other "managed" care programs, the Civilian Health and Medical Program of the Uniformed Services for military personnel and their dependents (CHAMPUS), care provided by the Veterans Administration (VA), employer-provided group plans, as well as government-allowed tax credits, deductions, and exclusions.[3]

All of these plans have, of course, been burdened by escalating costs, but those who rely on private insurance have been hit perhaps the hardest. In addition to general medical inflation, such plans are forced to pick up a portion of the tab for the uninsured and shortfalls in

From *Daedalus*, Vol. 121, No. 4 (Fall 1992), pp. 175–94. Copyright © 1992 by the American Academy of Arts and Sciences. Reprinted by permission.

Medicaid and Medicare reimbursement. As a result, premiums have often increased at two to three times the rate of inflation. Not that companies have not tried to cut costs, but all too often their strategies have very unfortunate consequences. We have seen that most private insurance companies, as well as many HMOs and Blue Cross/Blue Shield plans, now differentiate among health insurance applicants on the basis of expected health risk. Widespread screening increasingly leads to outright denials, exclusion of "preexisting conditions" from coverage, or exorbitant premiums for high-risk subscribers.[4] Small groups and individuals are the usual, but not the exclusive, targets of these practices; it is they who typically face experience-rated premiums (based on past sickness history) rather than community-rated ones (based on the average per capita costs of insuring a larger group).[5] Moreover, because a lost job may mean the loss of health insurance, even employees with good coverage fear the phenomenon of "job-lock," in effect becoming hostages to their current positions.[6]

Another strategy for cutting expenses is for employer plans and insurance companies to require increased copayments, coinsurance, and deductibles by patients. This not only shifts some of the financial burden to subscribers, but is theoretically supposed to encourage more frugal use of medical services. As an example of the growth of this trend, consider that in 1989, 17 percent of insured employees had plans with maximum out-of-pocket expenses of $2,000 or more; a year later, the figure had grown to 25 percent. Consider also that today over half of all group/staff HMOs require copayments (the patients' share of payments covered by insurance) for services.[7]

But efforts by insurance companies to control their own costs have not ended there. An enormously frustrating aspect of contemporary American medicine—for medical providers and patients alike—is administrative intrusiveness. Many insurance plans and HMOs routinely require costly utilization reviews that monitor providers' medical decisions, limit treatment, and constrain patients' choice of doctors and hospitals. The paperwork and second-guessing of physicians' judgments not only contributes to substantial and rapidly rising administrative costs, but confuses patients and angers their caregivers. One critic contends that such controls are "crippling the soul of the kind of doctor we should all want to preserve."[8] Indeed, 30 percent of physicians, according to one survey, say they would not have attended medical school if they had known what today's medical practices would be like.[9]

Although these alarming trends are not new, the hue and cry about them is. Complaints now emanate from all parts of the political spectrum. In a 1989 poll, 89 percent of Americans agreed that American medical care needs either "fundamental changes" or "complete rebuilding."[10] When a later Gallup poll posed the same questions to generally conservative chief executives, the figure was 91 percent. Indeed, few liberals would argue with the right-wing Heritage Foundation's conclusion that American medicine is critically ill and requires intensive care.

Certainly the extraordinary agreement on these ills—agreement across party, occupation, income, region, and age—represents a great opportunity for reform. Unfortunately, this "negative consensus," as sociologist Paul Starr has termed such broad dissatisfaction,[11] does not ensure that reform will be effective. Indeed, our politics, our institutions, even the ways in which the debate has been framed, make one fearful that the outcome will be quite the opposite.

FRAMING THE DEBATE

Classifying Reform Proposals

To facilitate intelligent debate about any subject, it is necessary to divide ideas and opinions into categories based on shared characteristics. Philosophers distinguish between "deontological" and "consequentialist" ethical theories; economists term macroeconomic theories "monetarist" and "Keynesian." In medical care, commentators generally divide major reform proposals into three groups, as discussed in Chapter 1: "play-or-pay," "single-payer," and "procompetitive."

Play-or-pay proposals would compel employers to provide health insurance for employees and their dependents, or pay a tax into a publicly funded plan to cover them. Businesses could either *play,* providing insurance that met certain minimum standards, or *pay* a tax, perhaps 7 to 9 percent of payroll, to support a government insurance program. In most play-or-pay schemes, the elderly, the poor, and the working uninsured would also be covered by this program, which would consolidate Medicare and Medicaid.

Single-payer proposals aim to provide universal coverage through a single government insurance plan. While there are a variety of such plans, the most widely discussed ones would attempt to adapt to the United States the key features of the Canadian system of insurance—a system in which doctors and hospitals are reimbursed from one insurance source, their provincial ministry.[12] In Canada, there is no private insurance except for those items not covered by the provincial plans (for example, dentistry, eyeglasses, and pharmaceuticals). As the sole

purchaser of medical services, provincial governments use their monopsony power to negotiate fee schedules with physicians (uniform rates
at which insurers reimburse providers) and global budgets with hospitals, including both operating and capital budgets. These periodic budget
negotiations tend to be noisy, contentious affairs—but unlike the negotiations of private insurance companies and providers of "managed
care" in the United States, they are out in the open for the public to
see and are subject to public influence through the political process.
The public is aware, after all, that it is financing the plan through
income, payroll, and sales taxes.

Wholly administered and largely funded by the provincial governments, Canada's universal health insurance permits a good deal of local
variation. The federal government does not prescribe the details of
provincial administration, but merely requires that provincial programs
embody the five basic principles of the Canada Health Act to receive
federal funding. These principles are as follows: programs must be
universal (covering all citizens), comprehensive (insuring all "medically
necessary" care), accessible to all (imposing no significant deductibles
or copayment obligations on individuals), portable (each province recognizing the other's coverage), and publicly administered (under the
control of a public, nonprofit organization).

The third type of reform proposal, procompetitive, explicitly rejects
the Canadian approach of controlling costs through negotiated budgets
for hospitals and fee schedules for doctors. Instead, these plans hope
to restrain medical inflation by fostering increased competition—between doctors, hospitals, and insurance plans. Since such proposals
promote private, rather than government, coverage, the problem of the
uninsured is seen principally as a financial one, a matter of giving those
without private insurance the financial wherewithal to purchase it. Tax
credits and vouchers are generally prescribed.

The classification of proposals into these three broad categories—
play-or-pay, single-payer, procompetitive[13]—is clearly useful in organizing the debate about medical care reform. There are so many plans out
there that we must group them in order to make sense of what would
otherwise be hopelessly confusing. And these particular classifications
are reasonable ones, highlighting important similarities and key distinctions among the various proposals. But if these classifications illuminate, they also obscure. Since classifications, by their very nature,
stress differences *between* groups and similarities *within* them, they
thus have a tendency to ignore their very opposites—that is, similarities
across groups and differences within them.

American politics has a way of exacerbating these inclinations. Take the case of abortion, where candidates and positions are labeled either "prochoice" or "prolife," even though this dichotomy obscures the reality that most Americans are, in effect, both. They want abortion to be legal and available, feeling that in some circumstances it represents a pragmatic, if tragic, way of dealing with an unwanted pregnancy. At the same time, most Americans are deeply troubled by abortion and want some regulations and restrictions on its availability and use—a waiting period, parental consent, limited public funding, stringent restrictions on late-term abortions, a ban on abortion for the purpose of sex selection. Few Americans support either the Democratic platform's position of "abortion on demand" or the Republican platform's stance that a fetus ought to be protected under the Fourteenth Amendment.

Whereas the abortion debate overemphasizes differences between groups, obscuring common ground, the debate over other issues stresses similarity within groups, clouding significant differences. Recall that Sam Nunn and Ronald Reagan were both supporters of the Strategic Defense Initiative (SDI) and thus were often portrayed as backers of "Star Wars," pure and simple. But what the classification blurred was the fact that while Reagan hoped for a space-based impenetrable shield that would ward off an all-out Soviet attack, Nunn thought such a system was unrealistic and destabilizing. Instead, Nunn favored a small, ground-based defense that would be effective only against a few missiles—perhaps an accidental Soviet launching, or an attack from a Saddam Hussein.

These same sorts of confusions permeate the debate about medical care reform. For example, some play-or-pay proposals would employ global budgets and fee schedules to control costs, just as Canadian-style single-payer plans would. But you would never know they shared these strategies from the intense focus on what they do not share. Moreover, if commentators often ignore similarities across groups, they also overlook differences within them. For instance, they talk and write about play-or-pay plans as though only one type of such a plan existed. As just noted, there are play-or-pay proposals that are designed to have global budgets and fee schedules to control costs, much like Canada; yet there are others that attempt to use the market mechanisms championed by procompetitive advocates.

A more important example of this tendency to stress similarities at the expense of differences is the failure to distinguish between two vastly different theories of procompetitive plans. One approach presumes that there is insufficient price competition in medicine and that first-dollar insurance (insurance, that is, without deductibles and cost-sharing) induces wasteful and financially costly patient demands. This view, which finds a home in proposals put forth by the Heritage Foundation and the Bush administration, argues that individuals should bear a greater share of their medical expenses and that doing so would encourage them to shop around for services and avoid needless care. The mechanisms for putting these policies into practice are increased deductibles and copayments, as well as the careful monitoring of medical services to counteract the fee-for-service incentives of providers.

By contrast, the "managed competition" approach, generally associated with Alain Enthoven of Stanford, rejects the notion that competition is feasible at the point of treatment. Enthoven argues that the "conditions under which the competitive market produces an efficient allocation of resources cannot be well satisfied by a market in which the 'product' the consumer buys is the individual medical care service."[14] He contends:

> First . . . If the insurance pays 80%, the consumer has an incentive to treat a unit of care that costs $10 as if it really cost $2. Moreover, in order to protect families from the risk of serious financial loss, an increasing number of insurance policies include an upper limit on the family's out-of-pocket cost above which all costs will be paid by insurance. At that point, the weak economic incentive introduced by coinsurance is removed altogether.
>
> Second, for most illnesses, the physician cannot quote a fixed price for treatment in advance. . . . Until he has done some work, he does not know whether you have indigestion or a heart attack. . . .
>
> Third, the individual episode of medical care is not good material for rational economic calculation. If the patient is in pain or urgent need of care, the transaction is not entirely voluntary. The sick patient is in a poor position to make an economic analysis of treatment alternatives or negotiate with the doctor over fees.
>
> Fourth, it is very costly for the patient to become well-informed about the costs and benefits of alternative treatments.[15]

All of this leads Enthoven to advocate competition among health plans rather than among doctors. Enthoven advocates empowering a small number of purchasing agents (large employers and state-created "public sponsors") to select a small number of insurance plans (most of which would be HMOs) among which its employees or "sponsees" must choose. Thus, although the Enthoven and Bush administration plans are both labeled "procompetitive," they in fact share little but the label.

Arguing Central Issues

Classification into basic types of proposals is not the only way in which the debate about medical care reform is framed. It is also commonly structured around certain underlying issues and principles. Chief among these are the questions of whether and how medical care should be rationed, the potential for eliminating waste and inefficiency in the provision of care, the use of competition versus regulation in controlling costs, and the often-asked question of whether there is a right to medical care.

Each of these four issues is important, some addressing profound philosophical concerns, others reflecting more mundane, but equally crucial, matters of policy. In discussion, however, much of their true significance is lost, since the issues are frequently posed in terms of oversimplified and misleading black-and-white choices. Frequently, too, these issues are used to call up ready-made emotional responses rather than to stimulate thought. Put another way, they are used like images of Willie Horton, and talk about "back-alley abortions," as symbols of what we fear most.

Rationing

In medical care, the most powerful image is that of rationing—an image generally called up by those who strongly oppose any government-run insurance scheme. The British National Health Service (NHS) provides the doomsayers' favorite illustration. As Canadian economist Robert Evans has noted, these critics depict "endless waits to see overworked and undertrained staff in obsolete and undermaintained facilities. Patients may even be denied lifesaving treatment if they are old or for other reasons fail to receive high enough priority for scarce services whose availability is controlled by heartless, or at least unaccountable, bureaucrats."[16]

Not only is the image of rationing fearful, but the word itself has powerful affective connotations. After all, when we think of rationing, we envision war—a time of death, destruction, and dire scarcity, when the government must, of necessity, strictly dole out meager supplies of life's essentials.

This is not to say that these images and connotations are without basis. Rationing can be a cruel and inefficient way of allocating scarce resources, as we have discussed in Chapter 6. But it is also, as any economist will note, one of only two ways of doing this. The other means of allocating goods and services is by price, a means which frightening images of rationing would seem to imply is benign. Of course it is not, as the 30 to 40 million Americans without health insurance, or the great majority of the rest who face copayments, deductibles, and excluded coverage can testify. Moreover, the problem of allocation cannot be perfectly solved, as some advocates of market-based medical care suggest, merely by ensuring that all have the financial resources to purchase comprehensive insurance policies. An immediate question arises: how comprehensive? Given that the government must inevitably assist in helping poorer subscribers in any such system, limits will be set. Will "comprehensive" insurance cover orthodontia, eyeglasses, pharmaceuticals, or psychiatric care for those who are apparently functioning members of society? Will it cover organ transplants—procedures whose mind-boggling fees for a single operation to possibly save a single life could clearly save more if spent elsewhere? Or will such services be allocated undemocratically, available only to those who can afford to pay for them on their own? The point is that whatever our medical care system—whether it allocates medical services primarily by price or by nonprice means—tough decisions have to be made as to who will have what and how much of it.[17]

Waste and Prevention

In answer to those commentators who focus on apocalyptic scenarios of rationing, some argue that difficult allocational choices can be avoided altogether if we would only eliminate inefficiency from our current arrangements, focus more energy on prevention, and all live healthier lives. As Joseph Califano, former Secretary of Health, Education, and Welfare has argued, "It is an unconscionable cop-out to resort to rationing by any means—the current scheme of wealth, or any new one based on age, a lottery of diseases or computer quantifications of pain—when we can have care for all our people with a little efficiency, prudence, and prevention."[18] But as wonderful as this you-can-have-it-all notion of medical care sounds, it turns out to ring quite hollow.

Let us begin with the concept of waste. The perpetrators are obvious:

excess capacity, useless bureaucratic hassle, medical malpractice, defensive medicine, not to mention the unnecessary tests and procedures resulting from all of this and on which most commentators tend to focus. In Chapter 5 a quotation from Edward Faltermeyer described a carotid endarterectomy as essentially an expensive "Roto-Rooter job." Other procedures are held in the same disdain.

Perhaps the medical profession does an inadequate job of evaluating the effectiveness of procedures. But there will always be procedures that, while of unproven benefit, nonetheless offer the possibility of help. And it is unlikely that any set of rules we design can significantly change this dynamic. However untested, therapies will always be sought by patients wanting to improve their lives, while doctors themselves will want to employ them. Monetary incentives certainly play a role, but physicians are also guided by a special professional ethic. Like lawyers who have a duty to do whatever it takes to serve their clients, doctors are committed to doing whatever they can to assist their patients. Absent a strong medical consensus as to the efficacy of a particular procedure—we rarely perform tonsillectomies any more, and radical mastectomies are increasingly open to question—there is little likelihood that either of the intimate partners in the doctor-patient relationship will ever perceive a significant proportion of medical treatments as "wasteful."

Now consider prevention. What if we all ate more wisely, exercised more regularly, abstained from smoking and excess drinking, and led less stressful lives? Certainly we would tend to be healthier; indeed, we might even be happier.[19] But the inference that we would, as a result, drastically reduce our national medical expenditures is, according to scholars who have investigated the possibility, without solid evidence.[20] The point is that prevention can, and has, changed the incidence of disease, but, at best, it can only delay death and dying. Indeed, although American preventive practices have served to improve our health record—and there is good evidence that they have, in the instances of heart disease and stroke—they have also brought onto the health policy agenda new issues of long-term care and frailty.

Competition versus Regulation

Both plans employing tax credits and vouchers and those promoting managed competition are labeled procompetitive. Advocates have carefully chosen this label so as to draw an explicit contrast with other approaches to universal health insurance. The implication is that the other proposals are not procompetitive, but anticompetitive and proregulation. But to present the choice facing us as that between competition and regulation is in a very real sense to set up a false dichotomy.

Note that managed competition plans backed by some procompetitive advocates favor competition that is far from unfettered—to the contrary, these plans necessitate extensive regulation, since they are hardly self-governing. For example, in the kind of competition between insurance plans encouraged by proponents of managed competition, some plans might thrive by only attracting and enrolling the young and healthy; while in rural areas, where it is often difficult to get even a single medical provider to cover the population, competition among plans, whatever the encouragement, might be totally infeasible. To avoid such imbalances, managed competition sets up detailed rules to govern the system. They require all citizens to enroll though specified purchasing agents in one or another of a limited number of preapproved insurance plans. For their part, participating insurance companies are forced to offer, not a single plan, but several predetermined varieties. But it is not only managed competition that is managed. Despite their procompetitive rhetoric, even more market-based reform proposals presume an extensive regulatory framework to combat market failures: the Bush plan forbade insurance firms from using experience-rating in pricing their policies; the Heritage proposal accepted experience-rating, but relied on state-regulated and administered insurance pools to cover high-risk individuals.[21]

The advocates of competition stress as well the rhetoric of free choice. For instance, Enthoven has labeled his procompetitive plan, described earlier, the "Consumer Choice Health Plan." As he explains: "The patient still has 'free choice of doctor' in the sense that he can join the health plan in which his favorite doctor participates. But now he also has the right to agree to get his care from a limited set of providers who offer him a lower premium and/or better benefits."[22] Not only is this a debatable notion of consumer choice—as Paul Starr points out[23]—but even if it were not, the idea of a favorite doctor is itself somewhat arcane. Could Enthoven himself tell us the name of his favorite otolaryngologist? How about his favorite gastroenterologist? And what is the likelihood that his favorite internist, cardiologist, neurologist, ophthalmologist, urologist, and proctologist are all members of the same health plan?

Enthoven seems to imply that Americans value the choice of an insurance company or health plan more than they prize the choice of a doctor. Surveys and common sense, however, both dispute this conclusion.[24] Consider the mind-set of someone faced with a choice between two health plans. One is a traditional Blue Cross/Blue Shield plan which allows unrestricted selection of physician and hospital. The other, an HMO, has lower premiums, but provides no reimbursement for physicians outside its network. Most people regard such a choice as burdensome, as being forced to opt unfairly for either money or the quality of their medical care. Clearly, this is not a straightforward "free" choice. Indeed, if the HMO is selected, the subscriber does not feel he or she has an enhanced degree of freedom, but rather has given up some of that freedom.

Is Medical Care a Right?

It is common for those who are deeply committed to reform but skeptical of its prospects to quip that national health insurance will only be possible when Americans overwhelmingly decide that medical care is a "right." It is not at all clear, however, that such agreement is a precondition for enacting universal health insurance.

To be sure, there is no evident consensus on medical care as a right. But almost all Americans agree that medical care should not be allocated primarily on the basis of ability to pay, and that everyone should receive a decent minimum standard of care. And they are right; medical care is no ordinary commodity. Not only is it, like food and shelter, a basic prerequisite for life, but the need for medical treatment is not just a matter of behavioral choices, but substantially a function of luck.

More generally, it is possible to reach agreement on health policy without having consensus on the justifying ideology. A social democrat may favor universal health insurance for purely egalitarian reasons, while a libertarian may support it on totally other, self-interested, grounds. Generally opposed to the expansion of government power, that individual nonetheless understands that if coverage is not comprehensive, those with insurance will inevitably have to pick up the tab for those without.

THE EFFECT OF POLITICS, INSTITUTIONS, AND IDEOLOGY

If the way the debate is framed hinders intelligent discourse and darkens the prospects for meaningful reform, so too does our politics. For one thing, the constitutional structure of our political system alone makes the process of legislative change difficult. As every civics book explains, it is designed for delay, not action, and characterized by myriad and conflicting governments—be they federal, state, or local. And where medical care reform is concerned, one must add to this maze an abundance of entrenched interests. After all, when $740 billion is spent annually on medical services, there are some big winners. The one unassailable law of health economics is that every dollar in expenditures is a dollar of somebody's income.

What our institutions make difficult, our ideological predilections make even more so. Historically, Americans have been fearful of concentrated authority and skeptical about government's capacity to manage public programs appropriately. So when Constance Horner, the Deputy Secretary of Health and Human Services until 1991, claimed that a national health insurance program run by the federal government would have "all the compassion of the Internal Revenue Service and the efficiency of the Postal Service, at Pentagon prices,"[25] her comment did not fall on deaf ears. Many Americans are worried about a government monopoly in the financing of medical care, and there are bases for the concern. Were national health insurance simply an enlarged instance of Medicaid, a poorly designed and managed program that ultimately pleases no one, it would indeed be disastrous.

Perhaps a more important ideological issue concerns taxes. To some, the antitax sentiment of the last 20 years is a demonstration of shortsighted greed and self-interest. Others see it as a healthy statement about the excess size, scope, intrusiveness, as well as limited competence, of modern American government. Either way, the sentiment is real, and it significantly affects debate on medical care reform. To many Washington politicians, any national health insurance program requiring a large tax increase is a nonstarter. To them, it is simply beside the point that increases in taxes for health coverage could well be more than offset by reductions in premiums for private insurance and out-of-pocket payments.

This institutional and ideological background leads many to conclude that any feasible reform must be incremental in nature. Our political system, entrenched interests, and antigovernment and antitax ideology simply do not allow for more drastic action. Not surprisingly, then, the overwhelming majority of reform bills in the House and Senate reflect this view, attempting to adjust our current arrangements in an incremental manner. On the Republican side, most proposals follow the Bush administration's plan of using vouchers and tax credits to give more individuals the financial means to afford more of the health insurance we now have. For the Democrats on the other side of the aisle, a number of their leaders—including President Clinton—also aim "to build on" our current system of employer-provided insurance. The more thoughtful advocates openly acknowledge that their stance is one of pragmatism. "The real problem with national health insurance," writes its long-time advocate Henry Aaron, a Brookings Institution economist who now argues for play-or-pay, "is the enormous disruption it would cause—including shifting more than $300 billion in financing from private payers to public budgets. . . . It is hard to imagine that American democracy, a system given to slow and incremental change, would embrace such a shift."

While the incremental approach may indeed be politically possible, it is characterized by significant drawbacks, most of them ignored by its advocates. Most obviously, any incremental reform will, by its nature, only be able to rectify some of the problems of the present system—though admittedly these are often very important ones. For example, many of the play-or-pay plans would for all practical purposes eliminate the problem of large numbers of uninsured. But while universal coverage is no small achievement, for the 85 percent of Americans who already have coverage, most play-or-pay plans would do little to address their complaints.

Another problem with incremental reform is that such plans fail to set up the kind of program architecture that can be built on. The experience of Medicare should alert us to the dangers this presents. In 1965, reformers like Wilbur Cohen and Robert Ball knew what they wanted eventually to achieve—a program covering care for all or most of the population—but concluded it was not politically possible at the time. Thus, they settled for hospitalization coverage for the elderly, assuming that Medicare benefits and eligibility would gradually expand. Hospital coverage was in their view simply the first step in benefits, the elderly merely the first group of recipients. Their optimism about future reform proved unrealistic, however, and twenty years later they regretted having left the system so vulnerable, so incomplete.[27]

The history of American government, then, suggests that the time to get the architecture of a program set is at the beginning, before benefits are expanded, not afterward. Concentrated interest groups are at their least powerful when the consensus on action is most firmly established. That was true in 1965, and it is why the Medicare reform of that year represents a missed opportunity. It is true now as well.

This highlights yet another risk of the incremental approach. A strong consensus provides a great deal of political capital, and reform, even when minor, spends much of it. This is especially true, given the tendency for reformers to believe they have been bolder than they in fact have been. The tax reform efforts of 1986 provide a case in point. Hailed at the time as an unprecedented, bipartisan step to close loopholes and simplify the tax code, it was soon after jokingly referred to as the "Lawyer Full Employment Act of 1986," having ironically made the code more complicated—at least until its often-vague provisions were clarified. Moreover, not only was the reform less effective and bold than advertised, but it made future efforts much more difficult: there was less public support for tax reform, and time was required for legislators to heal the wounds of having voted against the interests of various powerful constituencies.

THE PROBLEM OF IMPLEMENTATION

Henry Kissinger is fond of telling the following story. The President's National Security Adviser asks one of his top military analysts to develop a policy to deal with the problem of Soviet submarines. A few months later the analyst reports back to his boss, who promptly asks, "What is your recommendation?" "Heat up the world's oceans and boil the Soviet subs to the surface." "And how do you propose to implement this strategy?" questions the National Security Adviser. "Look," replies the analyst, "you asked me to come up with the policy— it's your job to implement it."

The efforts to classify and group reform proposals and the other ways in which the debate about medical care has been framed tend not only to block alternative perceptions of reform, but to obscure the all-important issue of implementation. After all, no one could intelligently argue that one plan is superior to another merely because it is play-or-pay as opposed to single-payer as opposed to procompetitive. To make evaluative judgments, one requires realistic forecasts of a plan's implementation and operation, whatever its basic approach.

Consider, for example, two proposals for American medical care, one a single-payer scheme, the other a procompetitive design. Both appear promising in theory, but the first, one surmises on the basis of its detailed features, is destined to become in practice a poorly structured, badly managed single-payer program—a kind of Medicaid writ large. The second, in contrast, has features that promise to work more effectively when implemented, resulting in a carefully and skillfully regulated program of managed competition, one where consumers choose from among a few high-quality, nationwide plans—much as they now do with long-distance telephone companies. No responsible advocate of Canadian-style, single-payer plans, however committed to government insurance, would favor the first proposal, given its practical ineffectiveness. Similarly, if we compare a well-worked-out single-payer plan with a poorly implemented procompetitive scheme, no thoughtful proponent of market-based reform would favor the latter, however intense her commitment to the theory.

It should be clear by now that any successfully implemented reform effort—whether single-payer or procompetitive, Canadian style or German style—will also require skilled government regulation and management. Yet this is often overlooked by advocates of all plans. On the one hand, procompetitive and play-or-pay advocates minimize the extent of government supervision required to make their plans work well. On the other hand, proponents of single-payer plans too often fail to address genuine concerns about the government's capability to manage such a system. Citizens cannot possibly watch the activities on Capitol Hill and feel fully comfortable turning over to Congress decisions on the resources available for medical care. Nor do Pentagon negotiations with defense contractors give one grounds for confidence in the government's talent in negotiating fees and budgets with doctors and hospitals. As for the savings and loan crisis, with its ineffective regulation of banking institutions, it hardly encourages trust in the government's ability to regulate health insurance plans.

But given the extent to which our politicians and policy analysts both enjoy abstraction and resist the difficult and unglamorous task of figuring out the nuts and bolts of real programs, this inclination to botch or overlook implementation is not very surprising. Nor is it simply a matter of intellectual failure. Our politics rewards superficial and generalized debate, name-calling, and symbol-rattling, rather than detailed analysis.

WHERE DO WE GO FROM HERE?

The problems facing us are serious and daunting. But we must proceed nonetheless. In which direction? Significantly, the two authors of this paper suggest different paths. Marmor encourages the pursuit of a single-payer plan modeled on the Canadian system. Boyum, in contrast, supports a form of managed competition, one that would completely sever the traditional linkage of insurance and employment, putting all citizens—whether employed, unemployed, or self-employed—on equal footing. Despite this, the authors agree more than disagree: on the diagnosis of the problems, on the necessity of systemic rather than incremental reform, and on the crucial importance of implementation.

It is our shared belief that a single-payer plan is unlikely to work well if managed within and according to existing government structures. What is needed instead is a strongly independent agency or government corporation set up—at a state or federal level—exclusively to manage the program, and well insulated from political pressures. We also agree that in the case of managed competition plans, successful realization depends on equally skilled government involvement, even though it would be of a very different kind from that required by a single-payer design.

Unfortunately, neither of us is sanguine about the prospects of achieving the kind of systemic reform for which both of us hope, whatever our particular preference. The likelihood is that our politics will leave Americans with confused choices, escalating inflation, and considerable despair. What is more, incrementalism would seem our destiny. But if so, we simply cannot leave it at that: the least we can do is distinguish between those strategies that do little more than tinker in an effort to patch up weaknesses in existing arrangements, and those that lead in the direction of fundamental reform.

Even this is not easy. For example, consider the long-awaited medical care reform proposal of the Bush administration, announced in early February of 1992. Although the proposal—which justly received few plaudits even from the conservative camp—was vague, poorly thought out, and deeply inadequate in its prescriptions, it nonetheless contained at least one remarkable feature. The proposal advanced the proposition that preexisting conditions and poor health histories should not be allowed to count in the price of health insurance, and that the costs of insurance should be spread widely, in the tradition of community rating. Importantly, such a step would go some way toward creating a more stable and more egalitarian insurance system.

Why did so few take note of it? For one thing, because of the sad but all too common tendency to overlook distinguishing and meaningful details of policy reform in the rush to facile judgment. For another, because to do so from the Left would be to give praise to the Right; while to do so from the Right would be to publicly accept some of the ideological principles of the Left. And unfortunately, our polarized politics too often precludes such generous admissions and reasoned assessments[28]—the very assessments needed to reach the common ground that would facilitate the enactment of effective reform.

Chapter 8
Reflections on the Argument
for Competition in Medical Care

WITH DAVID BOYUM

During the 1970s the discourse on American health policy shifted dramatically. The health debates early in the decade were marked by an atmosphere of urgency; indeed, the sense of trouble was so widespread that Republicans and Democrats, liberals and conservatives, competed over which form of national health insurance to offer in response. Perhaps more significantly, it was widely assumed that the necessary tools of reform were intensified planning and broader regulation. By the end of the 1970s, however, this approach had, for many, been discredited. To promarket advocates the answer was less regulation, not more, and competitive reforms became a dominant feature of health policy debate.

At least three factors made the increased attention to competition an understandable development. First, traditional concerns about access to medical care and the distribution of its costs began to take a back seat to worries about controlling the total cost of care. Problems of the uninsured and poorly protected could not compete for the public's attention with the genuinely ominous numbers on medical inflation. In 1970, the United States, possessing a strong and growing economy,

From Richard J. Arnould, Robert F. Rich, and William D. White, eds., *Competitive Approaches to Health Care Reform* (Washington, D.C.: Urban Institute Press, 1993). Reprinted by permission.

spent 7.4 percent of its GNP on health care. In 1980, with a weak economy still reeling from the twin oil shocks of the previous decade, the proportion was 9.1 percent.[1]

A second factor was the general ascendance, in academic writing, of economic approaches to analyzing public policy. Or more accurately, as Evan Melhado has pointed out, the ascendance of economic analysis that had a deregulatory mission.[2] Obviously the Chicago School comes to mind, but others who would hardly be associated with that movement, such as economist Charles Schultze and political scientist Theodore Lowi, were also influential.[3] All of this provided the intellectual groundwork for procompetitive health care reforms. Indeed, Melhado cites a personal telephone conversation in which "Alain Enthoven reports that he had read Schultze's book [*The Public Use of Private Interest*] shortly before devising his Consumer-Choice Health Plan and that he regards his [own] book as the 'working out' in the health care economy of an example of Schultze's general propositions."[4]

A third factor bolstering the competitive movement was the spread of such antigovernment, antiregulatory sentiment to the wider political arena. Although this has become synonymous with Ronald Reagan, it in fact had earlier roots. Americans often forget the extent to which Jimmy Carter ran for president on an anti-Washington, antigovernment platform, portraying himself as a down-home farmer who, pitchfork in hand, was headed to the nation's capital to slay the federal leviathan.

More than a decade after the 1970s, the intellectual themes of the health policy debate are remarkably similar. At the outset of the 1980s, many politicians and policymakers were looking to competition because health costs had soared to over 9 percent of GNP. Now medical spending absorbs something like 14 percent of our GNP,[5] and many are still looking to one or more of the many competitive approaches to health insurance and provision as the answer.[6]

To most of those who oppose competitive reforms, these numbers provide ample evidence that market forces simply cannot constrain health outlays. But the very same data on rising health expenditures are also presented as crucial evidence of the need for more competition—either among providers or among insurers—in American medical care. These advocates argue that a genuinely competitive market has never really been tried in the United States, and that our unabated inflation shows just how urgent the need for market competition really is. For example, in the 1991 survey of health care reform proposals by the *Journal of the American Medical Association,* Enthoven and Kronick argued that "contrary to a widespread impression, America has not yet tried *competition* of alternative health care financing and delivery plans, using the term in the normal economic sense, i.e., *price* competition to serve cost-conscious purchasers."[7]

They are quite right that a competitive market for health plans has never been implemented on a comprehensive scale. Instead, piecemeal, uncoordinated, and largely unsuccessful attempts have been made to introduce more competition into the delivery of medical services. A case in point was the invigorated application in the 1970s of antitrust law to the medical (and other) professions and the concomitant lifting of the ban on advertising.[8]

They may also be right that, if fully implemented, certain competitive systems, like Enthoven's Consumer Choice Health Plan,[9] would very likely restrain the growth of health care costs. It does not necessarily follow, however, that such competitive schemes are the answer to our medical care woes.

Many procompetitive advocates offer plausible, yet debatable, economic arguments to support their particular proposals. But intelligent policy ideas require a sound political grounding as well. Indeed, where medical care reform is concerned, any thoughtful policy analysis must address a whole host of issues, ranging from questions of political feasibility and practical implementation to concerns about distributional consequences and compatibility with professional ideals. It is to these matters that procompetitive advocates have generally paid insufficient attention.

PROBLEMS OF IMPLEMENTATION

Historical Evidence

In Chapter 7 we related an anecdote about policy implementation that is a favorite of Henry Kissinger. The point of that story was not to suggest that procompetitive reform proposals are as quixotic as plans to boil the oceans. Rather, the aim was to illustrate the need for policy ideas to have reasonable plans and prospects for implementation. Unfortunately for backers of procompetitive reform, historical experience—both international and domestic—is not reassuring.

On the international front, there is not a single country in the world to which procompetitive advocates can point as a model. They do, of course, use foreign medical care systems as negative models, as evidence of the failure of government-run insurance or care. But while it is undoubtedly important to examine and highlight the inadequacies of these systems, one must always be careful in comparing a hypothetical scheme (procompetitive) with actualized systems. As stock brokers and commodities traders often say, "Anyone can trade on paper."

By contrast, proponents of alternative strategies of reform—such as a single-payer approach—can look to a host of countries that provide their citizens with universal access to medical care at relatively low cost. Even more important, these policymakers can use international experience to help answer the most important of all implementation questions: how do we get there from here? After all, countries like Canada and Australia have fairly recently made the transition from a United States–style system to a single-payer design.

Nor should domestic experience make anyone hopeful about the prospects for procompetitive reform. Consider the case of HMOs, which many procompetitive advocates see as essential to combating the perverse incentives and informational asymmetries of fee-for-service medicine. Despite all the rhetoric about managed competition and legislative efforts to encourage the establishment and expansion of HMOs since 1973, only 15 percent of the U.S. population, or 36.5 million people, were enrolled in HMOs by 1990. One problem has been that throughout the 1980s HMOs and other managed care insurance plans failed to earn a reasonable rate of return. In 1989, 66 percent of established HMOs and only 46 percent of new HMOs were profitable. In both 1987 and 1988, HMOs reported average losses of over 4 percent on revenue; while 1989 showed an improvement, even in that year HMOs earned on average less than 1 percent on revenue.[10]

Another obstacle is that, plain and simple, doctors prefer fee-for-service. Eli Ginzberg suggests that many HMOs have been forced to rely on individual or independent practice associations, not on the pure HMO form as envisioned by Ellwood, Enthoven, and others.[11] This claim is backed by Marsha Gold's findings: "Network and individual practice associations (IPA)-model plans . . . increased from 97 to 433 between 1980 and 1990. Their share of HMOs increased from 41 percent to 76 percent, and of enrollment from 19 percent to 58 percent."[12]

The Need for Regulation

It is worth emphasizing that there are two broad theories of procompetitive reform, which we have explored in detail in Chapter 7. One approach presumes that there is insufficient price competition in medicine and that first-dollar insurance (insurance, that is, without deductibles and cost-sharing) induces wasteful and financially costly patient demands. This view argues that individuals should bear a greater share of their medical expenses and that doing so would encourage them to shop around for services and avoid needless care. The mechanisms for putting these policies into practice are increased deductibles and copayments, as well as the careful monitoring of medical services to counteract the fee-for-service incentives of providers.

By contrast, the managed competition approach rejects the notion that competition is feasible at the point of treatment. Enthoven we have seen, argues that the "conditions under which the competitive market produces an efficient allocation of resources cannot be well satisfied by a market in which the 'product' the consumer buys is the individual medical care service." He ends up advocating competition among health plans (most of which would ideally be HMOs) rather than among doctors.[13] Although they differ greatly in their theory of competition, both of these approaches employ the label "procompetitive."

Robustness

In arguing against government-financed or provided medical care, advocates of procompetitive reform often argue that governments are not sufficiently competent to manage such systems. For starters, it is claimed, the inevitable concessions of the political process ensure that, when finalized, policy programs bear scant resemblance to their initial design. Then inefficiency sets in, as governments are slow and ineffectual at responding to the results of their actions (which regularly include unintended consequences opposite to the intended ones).

Yet procompetitive advocates have proposed a variety of detailed government programs, laws, and regulations designed to address and eliminate the kind of market failures that might occur in unregulated medical markets. What happens when government incompetence contaminates these efforts? What happens to Enthoven's plan when only half of its provisions get enacted and implemented; when insurance companies are not required to offer specific types of plans; when the government increases, rather than eliminates, the tax deductibility of medical insurance? What happens if experience-rating is allowed, but the government sets up no provision for high-risk pools?

The answer may be that procompetitive plans are not robust, that they do not perform well unless conditions are just right. After all, by detailing those government actions required to eliminate current market failures, backers of procompetitive reform implicitly acknowledge that without these remedies, a competitive system does not work very well.

(Indeed, few would claim that our current system, plagued by skyrocketing costs and large numbers of uninsured, works well.)

ISSUES OF VALUES

Choice

In support of their policies, advocates of competition stress as well the rhetoric of free choice. Enthoven and others imply that Americans value the choice of an insurance company more than they prize the choice of a doctor. Surveys and common sense, however, both dispute this conclusion.

Access and Distribution

Few advocates of competition believe that medical care should be allocated solely on ability or willingness to pay. And their plans generally guarantee access to a "reasonable" or "decent basic minimum" of health care services. But at some point above this minimum, all procompetitive programs allow, and depend on, price-conscious behavior. In other words, they allow for some inequality of access or distribution based on willingness to pay.

As philosophers like Norman Daniels have illustrated, it is open to question whether such market-based plans meet the requirements of justice.[14] Nor is it clear to most Americans that a "decent basic minimum" is sufficient. A recent survey found that 91 percent of those Americans polled think that "everybody should have the right to get the best possible health care" and that 66 percent believe it unfair that some people can afford better health insurance than others.[15] And in spite of concerns over the cost of care, 63 percent in another survey favored making health care more available to everyone who does not yet have it rather than lowering the nation's health care spending.[16]

Professional Ideals

We have seen that despite the increasing rewards afforded American medical practitioners, they are increasingly dissatisfied. Because of managed care—an inevitable development under most procompetitive plans—doctors complain that they no longer enjoy the autonomy they once had. Rather, elaborate and expensive procedures, including utilization reviews, requirements for preadmission certification and other forms of second-guessing, have proliferated. AMA surveys found that 60 percent of physicians strongly oppose third-party reviews of their hospitalization decisions.[17] In a 1991 article in the *Atlantic,* Regina Herzlinger reported that more than 30 percent of current physicians say they would not have attended medical school had they known what their futures had in store.[18]

If doctors were concerned about these developments only to the extent that their incomes are threatened, we would not lose any sleep over it. But managed care has the potential to dramatically alter the relationship between doctors and patients; indeed, it already has. That relationship has always been considered special. It is not simply one of seller and buyer, or provider and consumer, as some economists crudely describe it. Doctors are asked to abide by a professional ethic to do whatever they can to assist their patients. And patients, who are at their physically and emotionally most vulnerable when they require medical care, expect this from their doctors. It is hardly reassuring for the patient to have his physician's medical judgment second-guessed (by his employer or insurance company) on grounds of cost-effectiveness.

CONCLUSION

It is not the purpose of this chapter to reject procompetitive approaches. Indeed, one of its primary themes is that issues of implementation are so important that no one could intelligently argue that one plan is superior to another simply because it is labeled procompetitive as opposed to, say, single-payer.

Many advocates of competition have thoughtfully diagnosed the various market failures that plague our current medical care arrangements. And many offer as well intelligent proposals to remedy these shortcomings. What this chapter asserts is that the arguments of most procompetitive reforms are, to date, inadequate. They too often fail to address issues of implementation, especially doubts about the government's capacity to do what their plans would require it to do. They also overlook important questions of whether their proposals are compatible with certain values—not just values of access and distribution, but also values of choice and professional ideals. Until advocates of competition address more thoroughly these political and philosophical questions, their analyses must be considered narrow and insufficient.[19]

Chapter 9
The Case for
Straightforward Reform

WITH CARLOS CANO

There is a remarkable consensus that the American medical care system needs a major overhaul. The critical unanimity on this point bridges almost all the usual gaps—between old and young, Democrats and Republicans, management and labor, the well paid and the poorly paid.[1] We spend more[2] and feel worse than our economic competitors, with nine out of ten Americans telling pollsters that health care requires substantial change.[3] This is the good news for medical reformers in the Clinton administration and the Congress.

The bad news is that, for a variety of ideological, economic, and institutional reasons, our politics have frustratingly failed to coalesce around a solution that satisfies the reasonable conditions for a medical care system worthy of a civilized society. Instead, the current proposals, with major backing by our politicians, are evasions of this civilized solution—wholly or partly unsatisfactory—and, if passed into law and practice, will soon require modification. Why can't we get on with what's necessary?

Reprinted by permission from *Arthritis & Rheumatism*, Vol. 36 (1993), pp. 1641–48, where it appeared under the title "The National Health Insurance Reform Debate: Will the Country Get What It Wants?" Copyright © 1993, American College of Rheumatology. An earlier version appeared as "Strong Medicine" in *Lear's*, Vol. 5, No. 12 (February 1993), pp. 18–22.

WHAT EVERYONE WANTS (WELL, ALMOST EVERYONE . . .)

What most citizens and many experts want from a modern system of medical care is not that complicated.[4] Nevertheless, many with vested interests will argue that what seems desirable is impossible:

> Universal coverage for all Americans, with no significant deductibles or copayment obligations.
> Universal insurance for all medically necessary care, free of complicated, "fine-print" exclusions and surprises.
> Freedom to choose one's doctors, hospitals, and individual treatment without bureaucratic hassles.
> "Portable" insurance, which follows the citizen and is not tied to a specific job or locale.
> Affordable universal insurance, which requires an overall budget limit, with clear public accountability for the balance among the obvious goals of easy access to health care, assurance of the quality of that care, and reasonable costs.

Every other nation rich enough to afford the benefits of modern medicine has come closer to meeting these needs than we.[5] Why is that?

WHY PEOPLE ARE BEFUDDLED AND ANXIOUS

Reformers of earlier periods—during the Progressive Era and the New Deal, under President Truman, and in the early 1970s—thought the passage of national health insurance was near.[6] They were bitterly disappointed. Then, as now, entrenched interests helped to block change by skillfully manipulating our fears and ideological beliefs to maintain the status quo. The medicoindustrial complex has repeatedly attacked national health insurance as a "foreign import," the government's "failed" answer to our medical woes that would reduce choice, increase costs, and destroy the quality of American medicine.

The Players in the Medicoindustrial Complex.   The key to understanding our health reform debate lies in an understanding of the economic stakes of modern medicine. Our national medical bill in 1992 was over $800 billion, more than $3,000 per American citizen.[7,8] As the late Senator Everett Dirksen used to say, "A billion here and a billion there and soon you're talking about real money." No one decides to spend that much on medical care, and no one sensibly claims we are getting our money's worth for those outlays. Rather, the total emerges from the millions of transactions among patients, doctors, hospitals, and insurers.

The one unassailable law of medical economics is that national health expenditures are equal to the incomes of those in the medical care industry. As a consequence, any effort to lower the costs of American medical care invites the fury of those whose incomes would suffer if cost control were successful.[9,10]

There is no mystery, then, about what the medical care industry stands to lose if citizens get what they want. The private health insurance lobby leads the opposition to national health insurance. Some $250 billion flows through their financial accounts as they take in premiums and distribute their share of the medical care dollar. Every one of those dollars earns income for the Aetnas, Travelers, and other giants of the for-profit insurance industry; the same applies to the nonprofit Blue Crosses and Blue Shields. Doctors receive less than 20 percent of American health care expenditures; however, doctors determine the expenditures for drugs, devices, diagnostic investigations, and hospitalizations. In the last decade, the fastest-growing sector of the medicoindustrial complex has been administrative.[11] Experts estimate that more than $100 billion is spent each year "pushing paper," marketing insurance plans, reviewing bills, collecting unpaid bills, and, most annoying of all to patients and physicians, precertifying, certifying, and postcertifying what procedures and costs the insurers will allow the doctor to perform and bill.[12]

What national health insurance promises is a limit on the fees doctors could charge and many, though by no means all, American physicians are alarmed by that prospect. As for hospitals, universal insurance would remove the problem of the indigent patient, but a limited hospital budget (or a rate-per-procedure) would undeniably constrain their financial leeway. What is more, a decent guarantee of coverage would limit private health insurance to the financing of amenities such as private rooms, and that would mean dramatic reductions in the funds the insurers would control.

Many physicians realize they could very well gain as well as lose from national health insurance. Their traditional spokespersons, however, emphasize future losses and, with practically unlimited budgets for lobbying and propagandizing, inundate our politicians, our newsrooms, and our televisions with fearful visions. Former President Bush was only repeating the industry's line when he claimed that national health insurance would have "the efficiency of the Postal Service, the warmth of the IRS, and the purchasing strategies of the Department of Defense."[13]

Why the Opponents of Reform Have Been So Successful in Shaping the Debate. Why, we might well ask, hasn't the medicoindustrial complex been denounced as the braying of the privileged? The reason is simple. With marketing skill, ample funds, and indifference to truth-telling regarding domestic and international experience, they have played to our deepest fears and beliefs and, in the process, frightened many of our political leaders. Consider the following everyday claims during the last presidential election.

Government-supplied health insurance, according to the repeated assertions of the insurance industry, would limit our choices and rob us of the benefits of the marketplace competition their industry provides. Canada's universal public health insurance may be acceptable there, they advertise, but Americans would never tolerate Canadian limitations: waits for nonemergency surgery, restrictions on charging more than the fee schedule allows, and so on. Seldom have such caricatures been distributed so widely so shamelessly, as any conversation with any Canadian official, liberal or conservative, will confirm.[14] But note the strategic assumptions of what can only be characterized as propaganda. The charges count on a reflex piety of Americans before our idols of "the marketplace" and "free choice." The charges ignore the fact that our "choices" under private health insurance are increasingly restricted, and the fact that a so-called free market in health care that gives advantage to the affluent is in conflict with our belief that medical services should not be allocated according to ability to pay.

The irony is palpable. The extra cost and complexity of our private health insurance industry might be justified if it gave Americans more choice in their care. In fact, it provides hassles, not choice. To businesses, health insurance benefits are an unpleasant problem; by 1990, U.S. corporations were spending more for health benefits than was retained as profits.[15] Patients want competent, responsive care; choosing among insurance packages, when employers make alternatives available, requires impossible calculations of the risks of different types of illnesses. It is not fun. It is doubtful that anybody, other than those whose salaries and profits depend on the present system, benefits from having many private insurers instead of one public insurer.

Opponents of government health insurance play on our fears of being trapped in a bureaucratic nightmare. They count on the absurd notion that bureaucracy is bad only when it is governmental, as though insurance companies were not bureaucratic. The American public, well tutored on this score, resonates all too quickly to any charge that government is inefficient. But polls tell us what the health insurance companies do not: namely, that Americans dislike insurance companies even more than they distrust the government. A majority of Americans, it is true, believe (inaccurately) that private health insurers are more efficient than their government counterparts. But the public regards private insurance as meaner, and prefers "bumbling bureaucrats" to "nasty insurers."[16]

Wasteful, unaffordable, and incompetent are other tags the medicoindustrial complex attaches to government health insurance. The rhetoric goes, "If you like the Postal Service and the savings and loan debacle, you'll love national health insurance." On reflection, however, the American medical care system is already like the savings and loan mess, which resulted from governmental *inaction*. The cure for our current medical care crisis, as in the savings and loan debacle, is for the government to take clear responsibility, not avoid it; to act, not to let the "market" work its will.

Moreover, if the post office were run like our medical "system," it would refuse to process mail for 35 million Americans and would require that others wait so long that their only alternative would be an expensive courier service. Our medical arrangement leaves millions uninsured and denies early or preventive treatment to countless others in circumstances where an ounce of prevention would be worth a pound of cure.

There is certainly cause for concern about the government's capacity to manage well. But this fact merely means that we need to attend carefully to the ways in which national health insurance is organized. The last two decades of government-bashing have numbed our sensibilities. We have many competent public institutions: the Federal Reserve Board, the Congressional Budget Office, and the Social Security Administration.

There is no more frightening image in American medical care debates than "rationing." The argument that national health insurance will reduce the quality of our medical services and, inevitably, lead to "rationing" proceeds from the bizarre notion that we do not currently ration care.[17] Every medical industry conference highlights the fearful future of "rationing by the government," playing on fears with impunity because the American public does not know, or cannot face, the reality that no medical care system can offer everything patients and doctors want or need on demand. (In other words, there is no escaping allocation of services; the real question is whether who gets what care when is determined by the seriousness of medical need rather than by the size of a patient's wallet.) In fact, American medical care is increasingly being managed and rationed outside the control of medical professionals. The rationing goes on mostly behind the scenes: in hospitals, clinics, the offices of preferred providers and health maintenance organizations, as well as in the millions of individual decisions not to seek care because of cost. As the *New York Times* announced in 1992, "Health care plans [are] cutting doctors' autonomy."

National health insurance would undoubtedly change the terms of rationing. Global budgets would limit funds, and allocational decisions would emerge from negotiations between medical providers and public authorities and within the medical profession. This situation would be difficult and at times acrimonious, but the procedures would be in the open and subject to public accountability.[18] In most of the Western world such processes have produced reasonable access to a full range of care in ways that leave most patients content with, rather than critical of, their medical care arrangements. It is hard to imagine how this form of "rationing" could be thought inferior to our current mix of indulgence and deprivation.

As for the expected loss of quality under national health insurance, what does this mean? If high-quality medicine means gourmet meals in hospitals, extensive cosmetic surgery, or the lavish use of expensive, high-tech diagnostic devices, it is not likely that a public program will pay. The segment of the population that now has easy access to such services would simply have to pay for them—just as in other national health insurance settings, from Canada to Scandinavia. If, on the other hand, quality means, for example, providing prenatal care to all expectant mothers, then universal health insurance will surely *improve* the quality of American medical care, reducing the costly high-tech treatment of newborns with preventable conditions.

Specters of losing our best doctors, as the propagandists tell us Canada has, further distorts the perception of "quality care" in a national health insurance setting. What these reports fail to mention is that Canada's ratio of medical applicants to medical school places is more than twice ours,[19] and their ratio of doctors to population is comparable to ours, with an overall rate of hospital and physician use per capita exceeding that of the United States.[20]

Opponents of national health insurance also count on our knee-jerk aversion to taxes in making their case. Other nations tax their citizens at far higher rates than we do, audiences are reminded. While spending 30 percent less per capita on medical care than we do, Canada taxes its most affluent citizens at rates of 40 to 50 percent. True—but not because Canadians spend more of their incomes on medical care. National health insurance would mean that medical expenses—now divided among the government, employers, private insurance companies, and patients— would be converted into public budget items. And American politicians would have to deal with the real issue of total costs and who bears them. Conveying this message to the citizenry is not impossible, but the political pattern of running against government, against tax increases, and for the wonders of the competitive market will have to be confronted.

Finally, there is the charge that national health insurance would be such a drastic change that our society could not process it. "The real problem," according to Henry Aaron, a longtime advocate of national health insurance who doubts its current feasibility, is "the enormous disruption [national health insurance] would cause—including shifting more than $300 billion in financing from private payers to public budgets." According to Brookings economist Aaron, "It is hard to imagine that the American democracy, a system given to slow and incremental change, would embrace such a shift."[21]

The relevant question, however, is who would pay more or less for medical care, rather than what one calls the payment. Whether Aetna or Medicare channels the funds to medical care providers is unimportant to those Americans. What the public really dislikes is high personal taxes. High corporate taxes are, if anything, popular. A corporate tax that simply took from companies what they are currently paying for insurance would go unnoticed by the public. As for the corporations, they don't like taxes, but they don't enjoy paying for insurance either. Lower administrative expenses and a reasonable prospect of better control of future costs seem more favorable than an extension of the status quo. But without political leadership on explaining the realities of how we pay for care, the aversion to taxes will cripple our capacity to choose wisely.

Troubling questions about any shift to national health insurance are easily raised, but the public should be skeptical of the skeptics. The aim is to create a health insurance program that is successful, not perfect. We should not be misled by the "nirvana fallacy"—that we have already achieved, or are about to find, perfection. According to the *New York Times,* perfect bliss lies in an untried method called "managed competition." The current system is not working, and most people know it. We have tried incremental tinkering with "market reforms" for the past two decades, with far too little success. Our political leaders need to explain why our incrementalism has failed to work in a way that demonstrates that national health insurance would work better.

DOING WHAT'S RIGHT, WHAT'S NECESSARY, AND WHAT'S EFFECTIVE

If the way our medical care debate has been framed hinders intelligent discussion and darkens the prospects for meaningful reform, so too does our politics. Our constitutional arrangements alone make the process of legislative change exceedingly difficult.[22] As every civics book explains, American government is designed for delay, not action. Where medical care is concerned, entrenched interests are pressing to keep their portion of this huge feast. The winners at this table have no inclination to give up their gains or positions quietly.

What our governmental institutions and medicoindustrial complex make difficult, our ideological predilections make even more so. Historically, Americans have been fearful of concentrated authority and skeptical of government's capacity to manage public programs appropriately. Many Americans worry about a government monopoly in medical care financing, and there are real bases for the concern. Were national health insurance simply an enlarged form of Medicaid, it would be disastrous.

The antitax sentiment of the past 20 years is an even more important constraint on our choices. To some, the hostility toward increased taxation is a sad demonstration of shortsighted greed and self-interest; to others, it is a healthy and helpful statement about the excessive size, scope, intrusiveness, and limited competence of modern American government. Either way, the sentiment is real, and it affects our debate on reform. To many Washington politicians, any national health insurance program requiring a large tax increase is a nonstarter; it is beside the point that increases in taxes for health insurance coverage could well be more than offset by reductions in premiums for private insurance and out-of-pocket payments.

This familiar background leads many to conclude that any feasible reform must be incremental. Our political system, the entrenched interests, and antigovernment and antitax ideology, they contend, simply do not permit more fundamental change. Not surprisingly, then, the overwhelming majority of reform bills in the last Congress reflected this view, proposing to adjust our current arrangements piecemeal. On the Republican side, most proposals—including that of former President Bush in February 1992—offered vouchers and tax credits to give more

Americans financial assistance in buying more of the health insurance we now have.[23] For the Democrats, a number of their congressional leaders proposed reforms that "build on" the existing system of employer-financed health insurance, advocating the so-called play-or-pay plans.[24]

While a step-by-step approach has some obvious political advantages, it has great drawbacks to which proponents seldom draw attention. Incremental reforms by their very nature address only some of our medical care problems. For example, many of the play-or-pay plans would, in practice, eliminate the problem of the uninsured. No mean achievement, one would rightly say. But universalizing insurance would not address the complaints of the 85 percent of Americans who already have coverage.

Another serious problem with an incremental approach is its failure to take seriously the need to change the basic rules of the medical finance game while the window of political opportunity exists. The experience with Medicare should alert us to the danger of missed opportunities. The reformers of 1965 assumed that Medicare was but the first step toward universal public insurance. On that optimistic assumption, they were willing to settle for 60 days of hospitalization coverage for Medicare's elderly beneficiaries. Hospital coverage, in their view, was simply the first step in benefits, the elderly merely the first group of recipients. Such forecasts turned out to be extraordinarily mistaken and, nearly 30 years later, many regret our having been so cautious at the outset.[25]

American governmental arrangements suggest that the time to get the architecture of a program set is at the beginning. Powerful interest groups are least influential when consensus on reform is most firmly established. That was true in 1965, and explains why Medicare represents a missed opportunity. It is true now as well. The consensus on the need for change is like political capital, and any reform, even when minor, spends much of it. This is all the more important, given the tendency of reformers to regard themselves as being on the frontiers of possibility.

The Clinton administration is unlikely to take incremental steps. As Clinton fully noted in the campaign of 1992, increasing insurance in the absence of reliable constraints on cost would worsen the very medical inflation that has prompted much of the movement for reform. What the Republicans offer as anti-inflationary medicine is palpably defective. They blame medical inflation on misguided patients who are overinsured at work, and they presume that increased cost-sharing by the patient will produce the right mix between need and treatment. And they hope that "managed care" will do the rest. Growth in patient cost-sharing and programs of managed care over 20 years has not proved successful and is ample reason to reject this approach.[26]

THE REFORM AGENDA IN 1993

Clinton's presidential victory suggests that Americans are at least open to the idea that government may be able to do something they want done, and do it well. Even so, many of our politicians seem reluctant to set their sights on a health insurance system ambitious enough to deliver what it promises. A few cling to play-or-pay plans because they appear incremental, building on the image that mandated insurance does not "tax" workers. Others forsake caution for radical (even utopian) optimism, backing managed competition, as the *New York Times* incessantly claims, because, although untried and untested, it is the very "best plan for health care reform."

Managed competition appears to offer a political free ride. It preserves the illusion of a self-regulating market in health care, leaving the crucial decisions in the hands of private actors currently known as health insurance purchasing cooperatives. But neither play-or-pay nor managed competition alone will deliver what is wanted. Not that taking care of our health finances properly will be easy, as the experience of Canada and the other industrial democracies shows. National health insurance is no panacea. The trouble is that the other proposals for providing decent, accessible, portable, accountable, and affordable medical care are less satisfactory.

In 1991–1992 play-or-pay was the most widely discussed of these plans. It would mandate health coverage for all by requiring every business either to provide insurance for its employees or to pay a premium into a public fund, administered by government, for the benefit of everyone not covered at work. But no slogan, even an athletic and financial metaphor like play-or-pay, can disguise the fact that most variants of this approach seem designed to enable politicians to evade two hard truths.

The first is that medical care has to be paid for, and when the government "mandates" anything that costs money, the payment deserves to be called a tax. Play-or-pay is a fig leaf over this incontrovertible fact, but no one will be fooled for long. The second trouble with play-or-pay is that it tries to preserve a market in insurance plans while claiming to provide what no such market can provide without complex regulation and cross-subsidies: equal access to insured care regardless of ability to pay and medical status. Offering employers a choice between private and public plans threatens that the public plan will become a dumping ground for the worst health risks, a default position with the highest per capita costs. The only way to avoid this outcome, and with it a bitterly invidious two-tier health system, would be for the government plan to compete in quality and cost with the employer plans and to monitor retrospectively the risk selection of the competing plans. But this would reinsert national health insurance and the very government taxes and regulation play-or-pay was designed to avoid.

Play-or-pay is a sheep in sheep's clothing, but managed competition is a wolf in sheep's clothing. As touted in the *New York Times,* managed competition is a plan under which "large groups" of consumers will seek out, or be sought out by, "sophisticated sponsors" who would represent them in negotiations with insurance companies, doctors, and hospitals, "forcing" these providers to offer "high-quality treatment at reasonable cost." These sophisticated actors might be entrepreneurs, businesses, groups of businesses, unions, professional organizations, and the like. But whatever they are, they would have the clout to "manage" both needy consumers and greedy providers.

There is a powerful element of radical paternalism in the managed competition idea, which aims to do for everyone—doctors, patients, drug firms, and insurers—what is good for them, all in the name of controlling costs. The end result would be the sort of "managed care" arrangements with which we are already familiar—health maintenance organizations, preventive care group practices, and the like—but writ large. Rather than just setting ceilings and rates, such plans presume to make decisions in individual treatment. They ignore the fact that Americans dislike being "forced" or "managed" to do anything; they ignore as well that health maintenance organizations and their variants guarantee the rise of large private bureaucracies which themselves increase both costs and administrative complexity. Even more, the administrators of these systems would be tempted to put considerations of cost above quality of care. Governments would be tempted to do the same, of course, but unlike the "sophisticated sponsors" of managed care, would have to answer publicly if and when they succumbed to the temptation.

There is at least an ideological argument (the preference of marketplace competition) for the status quo over national health insurance. One can make a moral argument, in terms of widened access, for play-

or-pay over the current system. But once one rejects the market arguments, as Joseph White of the Brookings Institution has said, "there is
no case, ideological, moral, or practical for choosing play-or-pay or
managed competition over national health insurance" (personal com-
munication). What remains is only the political fallout of the fears and
befuddlements we have outlined: a compromise of what is desirable to
arrive at with what seems doable.

The task for reform is to show that what is desirable is in fact doable.
And to accomplish that, we must be clear about what national health
insurance has achieved in political and economic circumstances similar
to our own. The example of our Canadian neighbor, as *Consumer
Reports* demonstrated in a remarkable series of articles during the summer of 1992, is where we should look for evidence.

The Canadian model of national health insurance has been, for a
couple of years now, the object of extensive commentary. But it could
not possibly be accurately understood from the mix of myths, half-
truths, and misleading evaluations that the special-interest groups in
American medicine understandably express and to which the media
give excessive attention. The problem is that the truth about Canada is
moderately complicated, the health pressure groups have little interest
in accuracy, and few media outlets are capable of conveying the complexity.

Boldly stated, Canadian national health insurance has removed medical care from the ordinary processes of commercial markets. It has by
and large distributed care according to the seriousness of the illness,
not the thickness of the pocketbook. It has substituted the concentrated
interest of public officials for patients and health insurers as the nego-
tiators of payment. Canada uses government—as a kind of consumer
cooperative—as the vehicle for balancing the never-ending wish for
more care with the necessary discipline of an overall budget. And it has
done so over the past 20 years with considerable success, covering
every Canadian man, woman, and child while spending about 30 percent
less per capita than we pay for incomplete, complicated, and uneven
health insurance protection.[27]

Nothing about the Canadian means to these results is impossible to
outline. The striking aspect of the Canadian system is that its operational
principles are straightforward and intelligible to any citizen. Those principles discipline the national health insurance program in useful ways.

Everyone is in the same boat, which is what the principle of universality requires. All medical care that physicians can defend is open to
reimbursement, meaning its benefits are "comprehensive." The policy

applies wherever you are in Canada—that is what "portable" means. There is in every province a responsible political authority which has to answer for the trade-offs among quality, cost, and access—that is what "political accountability" means. And there are no complicated arrangements for cost-sharing by sick people (deductibles, coinsurance)—which is what is meant by "no financial barriers to care."[28]

It is easy to see why there is tremendous pressure to weigh policy changes carefully. With everyone in the same boat, the interests of the politically powerful are intertwined with those of the less articulate, and all of this helps to explain both the contentiousness of Canadian debates about cost and care and the high levels of satisfaction Canada's citizenry enjoys. It does not mean national health insurance is easy to enact or to manage. Nor does it mean that the United States could borrow wholesale the details of Canadian administration. But the argument that national health insurance in North America is impossible is *itself* implausible.

It would be foolish to ignore the Canadian experience, just as it would be foolish to try to replicate it in every detail. What we learn from Canada—and from Australia, Sweden, France, West Germany, and every other industrial democracy—is that an aroused public, aided by energetic political leadership, can extend the frontier of the politically possible and make national health insurance work. To make it work is not to have the fantasy of a self-regulating system that never needs adjustment. But that we should harbor the hope for a decent form of national health insurance in the near future is utterly reasonable. It is ethically and financially desirable, politically possible, and administratively implementable. But the opportunity will not come again soon.

Chapter 10
The Missing Alternative:
How Washington Elites Pushed
Single-Payer Reform Plans off the Agenda

WITH TOM HAMBURGER

In February 1993, Quentin Young flew to Washington from his home in Chicago, pleased to have been asked to consult with top White House officials on health care. Young, the past president of Physicians for a National Health Program, was looking forward to plumping for his organization's favorite cause: adapting Canada's national health insurance system to the United States.

Young had an attractive case to make. Canada, where provincial governments act as single insurers, annually spends 30 percent less per capita than Americans do for health care, providing universal coverage, cost controls, and choice of physician. The United States fails to insure 37 million people and has no control over rising costs. A Harvard University survey of ten nations found that Canadians were the most satisfied with their health care system; Americans were the least.

But Young's enthusiasm quickly withered within the White House

Reprinted by permission from *Washington Monthly* (September 1993), pp. 27–32. The article was published under the title "Dead on Arrival: Why Washington's Power Elites Won't Consider Single Payer Health Reform." Copyright © The Washington Monthly Company, 1611 Connecticut Avenue, N.W., Washington, DC 20009.

Tom Hamburger is the Washington Bureau Chief of the *Minneapolis Star Tribune*.

gates. It turned out, in Young's words, that he had been invited for "pseudo consultation." White House staff members made it clear that single payer was off the table. "Why?" Young asked, amazed. A senior White House health adviser, Walter Zelman, put it bluntly: "Single payer is not politically feasible."

In a separate session with Hillary Rodham Clinton, David Himmelstein of Harvard Medical School (a close colleague of Young), also pressed the single-payer point. Canada's solution, he said, made sense for the United States. Himmelstein has shown that this country could save as much as $67 billion in administrative costs alone by cutting out the 1,500 private insurers and going to a single government insurer in each state—easily enough money to cover every uninsured American.

Hillary Clinton had heard it all before. How, she asked Himmelstein, do you defeat the multibillion-dollar insurance industry? "With presidential leadership and polls showing that 70 percent of Americans favor [the features of] a single-payer system," Himmelstein recalls telling Mrs. Clinton. The First Lady replied, "Tell me something interesting, David."

So by February, fewer than six weeks into the Clinton presidency, the White House had made its key policy decision: before the Health Care Task Force wrote a single page of its 22-volume report to the President, the single-payer idea was written off and "managed competition" was in. But why should an intelligent First Lady and her 500 health care advisers *not* want to debate every option, especially examples available from nations that have combined universal access and cost control?

Because in Washington's political culture incremental change is the coin of the realm, and a move to single payer is seen as anything but incremental. (Though in fact, managed competition proposes a more drastic shift in health care delivery for most Americans than single payer does.) "I've been in so many meetings in Washington where people say, 'We've got to fashion something that's acceptable to the interest groups,'" says Minnesota Senator Paul Wellstone, one of the few single-payer champions. "And I know what groups they put at the top of the list—the health care and insurance lobbies." But there's more to the failure to discuss single payer than lobbyists and their clout. Some politicians fear being caricatured as advocates of "big government" in an age of sound-bite politics. And some fear being dismissed as irrelevant for supporting a cause that is thought to be outside the mainstream. What constitutes the mainstream? To understand that, consider the capital's three established tribes—the politicians, the press, and the experts—and how they slid single payer off the table.

First, politicians like Mrs. Clinton fear the bitter, unique opposition of the health insurance industry to single payer. Doctors, hospitals, and health insurers will oppose elements of any reform, but only a single-payer plan means the virtual abolition of an entire industry as we know it. Politicians who are reluctant to take on established interests in Washington ($60 million in medical and insurance Political Action Committee, or PAC, contributions since 1980) and back home (insurance agents in every Rotary Club in every district) are terrified by the anger that would result from putting health insurers out of business. Combining this with the normal opposition any reform provokes and with a political process that discourages full debate, politicians duck the merits of the issue and dismiss single payer as not feasible.

Once this political fact has been established in the hearts and minds of politicians, the people who might be expected to raise out-of-the-mainstream questions—reporters—are generally too focused on politics, not on substance, to do anything more than reflect prevailing opinion rather than informing it.

Finally, the experts who might be expected to rise above the political currents resist seriously appraising Canada for fear of being dismissed as cranks or out of touch with realpolitik. Those experts who *do* argue for single payer are penalized by having to chase research dollars with more difficulty at foundations where insurance executives are a presence. And so it is that an industry which employs 140,000 people in the United States helps kill reform that would help 250 million Americans.

There is the human drama, too, of watching these tribes operate in unhealthy symbiosis. Once something is thought to be off the agenda—as single payer has appeared to be—then it is death for a Washington player, no matter how established, to keep banging away. Take Congressman Jim McDermott, a Seattle Democrat, who despite years of talking up single payer still feels the sharp dismissiveness of his colleagues and understands why so few people challenge the status quo. A few months ago, McDermott and the rest of his state's congressional delegation won the coveted invitation to fly with Clinton on Air Force One to the Pacific Northwest's timber summit. In that collegial atmosphere, at the center of power, the politicians congregated around the President in his cabin.

McDermott raised his hand, and everyone groaned. "He's going to ask about single payer again," they muttered. He wasn't, but it didn't matter. "You get stereotyped and people act like they know what you're thinking and they become dismissive without listening to what you have to say," claims McDermott, a psychiatrist who came to Congress in

1988. "You have to put up with a certain amount of ridicule. This is an issue on which everybody has an opinion. And if you choose the wrong solution, you can be defeated."

The word is out among Democrats in the capital: positions like McDermott's, which appear to contradict the Clintons' approach, are considered disloyal to the new President. More to the point, the conventional wisdom goes, *why* would any halfway savvy Washingtonian want to fool with something that's off the table? Among the politicians and the press, where does this conventional wisdom begin to form?

Welcome to the world of the Sperling breakfast group. In the understated elegance of the Sheraton Carlton Hotel, two blocks from the White House, Washington reporters meet several times a week with prominent news sources. The event, hosted by the *Christian Science Monitor*'s Godfrey Sperling, Jr., recalls an older, more genteel era in Washington. Old in style, the setting reflects the continuing nature of most Washington journalism—reporters transcribing the thoughts and words of highly placed sources.

Senate Majority Leader George Mitchell dropped by one of these gatherings in July. Even before the waiters brought out the bacon and eggs, the questioning turned to health care: Do you favor consideration of Canadian-style health reform, the most popular solution among your constituents in Maine?

"No," Mitchell said bluntly. Canada's system may be good for Canada, but "it will not be enacted" in Washington. Americans want an American solution (a phrase Mrs. Clinton would also use during her working July holiday in Hawaii, sitting poolside with reporters). A couple of months before, when Mitchell met with the *Wall Street Journal*'s lunch group at the same hotel, he outlined the key elements he would like to see in a reformed American health system. His answer was crisp and precise: insurance coverage for all, controlled costs, consumer choice of physician and hospital, renewed emphasis on primary over specialized care, and flexibility for states to tailor the plan to their own needs—all of which perfectly describe the Canadian plan.

When pressed on the point, Mitchell said, "I respect the Canadian system . . . but we ought to select the system that's based on the practices and standards of our country. When very wealthy people— kings and prime ministers and others of means—in other countries get sick, they don't go to Canada. They don't go to Germany. They don't go to Japan. They come to the United States." Reporters at the Sheraton dutifully recorded Mitchell's words. Never mind that foreign leaders regularly use their own systems in Germany, Japan, Canada, and elsewhere. Never mind that just a few years ago Mitchell's Senate colleague, the late Spark Matsunaga of Hawaii, went to Canada for new, high-tech cancer treatments that were unavailable in the United States.

With such broad agreement on what health reform should provide, why don't the Canadian or the German or the Australian systems get more seriously considered? The short answer is fear. For politicians, this means mostly fear of political attack, fear of taking on powerful American myths, and fear of incurring the wrath of the well-endowed health care and insurance industries. And politicians fear being left out of the game. That means they talk the prevailing talk and think the prevailing thoughts, instead of realistically appraising proposed reforms or genuinely evaluating foreign experience.

Mitchell is well aware of the power of advertising to defeat single-payer advocates. His Republican colleague from Maine, Senator William Cohen, beat a Democratic challenger in 1990 in the nation's first election to turn almost entirely on health reform. Cohen's opponent, Neil Rolde, openly championed the Canadian-style system, but Cohen's campaign was guided by Republican pollster Bill McInturff, a clever conservative with an uncanny knack for packaging effective attacks.

"We trashed the hell out of the Canadian system," McInturff recalled. Foreshadowing the tack Bush took in his own reelection campaign, McInturff described how he planned ads attacking national health insurance with footage of a crowded Department of Motor Vehicles waiting line. The ominous voiceover? "This is your health care system if we go to a national plan." McInturff's GOP strategy rightly assumed that voters associate Democrats with big government, high taxes, and bureaucratic hassles. So McInturff shrewdly responded to a Democratic national health proposal by raising the specter of big government run amok, linking Canada with this dismal image. And McInturff was among those who recommended the line that Bush would later use in 1992 about how government health insurance would combine the efficiency of the postal service with the compassion of the KGB.

Clinton, as usual, was a step ahead of Bush—and, by extension, of McInturff. In the Democratic primary campaign, Clinton regularly referred to what we could learn from the experience of other nations. But in the general election campaign, Clinton suddenly adopted the phrase "managed competition" to define his variant of health insurance reform. Few understood then or now what he meant, but no one—especially political or industry opponents—could accuse him of foisting "failed" foreign ideas on the good old USA.

The institutional pressure on politicians to play it safe is powerfully dramatized in the cautious attitude of a reformer elected with Clinton: Congressman Bobby Rush of Chicago. In 1992 Rush, a former Black Panther, campaigned as an advocate of Canadian-style reform. Once introduced to the pressures of Washington, his former supporters claim he became skittish about cosponsoring a single-payer solution. Rush shocked Quentin Young and others by refusing to cosponsor Jim McDermott's single-payer bill in the House. Rush told supporters, including Young, that as part of the leadership (House Speaker Tom Foley had made Rush a freshman whip) it would be difficult for him to support a nonadministration bill, and that important supporters (medical, hospital, and insurance PACs donated $13,750 to Rush's campaign) would also not understand if he went along with the single payers. Outraged Chicago health activists who had supported Rush pressed him hard, and eventually he signed on. A Rush spokesperson says that Rush was just being "deliberate" as he considered a complex subject and did not delay because of other pressures. But when the tribal need to be accepted as part of the system is so strong that someone like Rush hesitates, it is little wonder that politicians of lesser proven conviction slip so readily into complacency.

NO, CANADA

So if politicians fear treading in the single-payer arena, why aren't journalists learning and talking about Canada and other foreign experience? Why are discussions of these matters relegated to largely arcane academic journals and occasional features? To be sure, there are thoughtful mainstream pieces from time to time. In July of 1993 the *New York Times* ran a detailed article explaining the advantages of Ontario's system of caring for the elderly. The *Philadelphia Inquirer* ran an extensive three-part series the previous April comparing Canadian, German, and American patient care.

But most of the time, almost any news story in Canada about waiting lists, a disappointed physician, or the lack of funds for doctors or hospitals finds its way into congressional testimony and into American news stories. Medical pressure groups do the digging and journalists do the disseminating. Because America's journalistic ethic of quoting both sides gives equal space to those who praise Canada and those who criticize it, articles repeat myths about Canada without analyzing them.

For example, in March 1993 the *New York Times* ran a major front-page piece headlined "Patients Footing the Bill amid Canadian Cutbacks: Spending Outstrips Government's Ability to Pay." Beyond that alarming head there was quite different news: the Canadian system is widely popular and 95 percent of all Canadians reported receiving the care they needed within 24 hours. The cutbacks? The Canadian government had decided not to reimburse its citizens any longer for electrolytic removal of unwanted hair.

A search of 100 health care articles in the *Washington Post* since April found that only 10 percent dealt substantially with Canada; 70 percent focused on leaks from the Health Care Task Force and on the political implications of the Clinton plan. Only three focused critically on managed competition. A cover story in the *Post*'s health supplement in June trumpeted a financial crunch hitting Canada's system. The cover art? Bill and Hillary as Adam and Eve in a health care Garden of Eden looking at a half-eaten Canadian apple. The headline? "The Model Is Tempting, But . . ." The lead? Canadians "know well how expensive it is to run a national system with universal coverage: they have one and evidence is mounting that they can't afford it." This makes little sense. Costs have risen over the past decade in Canada, but at nowhere near the rate U.S. costs have. So if we have nonuniversal coverage and spend 14 percent of GNP, how can a system with universal coverage that costs 9 percent of GNP illustrate the point that Canadians "know well how expensive it is to run a system with universal coverage"? Viewing the United States from Canada reveals exactly the opposite. It shows how expensive it is *not* to have universal coverage and cost constraints.

Why do such items get into print? First, there is the matter of sophistication. Few American journalists spend enough time studying the health systems of other developed democracies to know that the lessons thought peculiar to Canada are in fact quite general. Germany, France, Japan, Australia, and Canada all combine universal coverage with budget limits and considerable bargaining power in the hands of payers. Second, there is the matter of drama. (In mainstream journalism, bad news is always more interesting than good news.) So for dramatic reasons, even when stories explaining the benefits of Canadian or European systems do appear, they tend to be underplayed. For example, when the Congressional Budget Office (CBO) reported in May 1993 that a single-payer system could provide universal health care and still cut costs by $14 billion a year, the *Post* ran a single-column story inside the paper that never referred to Canada. A second CBO report in July saying that a Canadian-style plan would save more money than any other proposal—including managed competition—ran on page A15.

There are other factors at work here, too. Even after Watergate and

Iran contra, journalists are still reluctant to challenge the statements of public officials. During the 1992 campaign, for example, candidate Paul Tsongas flatly dismissed the idea of national health insurance. Dramatically, Tsongas said he might be dead today if he had been living in Canada, because the medical technology that saved his life from cancer was unavailable there. But it was not true. In fact, the treatment Tsongas needed was developed by Toronto doctors and is available to Canadians with little or no delay from the surgeons who helped invent it. At the time, most reporters never bothered to check on whether Tsongas' remark was true; the *New Yorker* and the *Chicago Tribune* followed up and told readers that a major presidential aspirant didn't know what he was talking about.

Why aren't more reporters and news organizations examining the system for themselves? Why do they fail to investigate exaggerated complaints and underplay positive reports? They aren't corrupt or being bought off by the insurance industry. The more compelling explanation is less scandalous, but more serious. Over and over again, reporters hear that the Canadian system "is not politically feasible." Over and over again, they hear that Canada is not the perfect system advocates make it out to be. These messages do not come solely from the spoonfeeding at lunch and breakfast meetings. Most important, once health care becomes a political issue, it is assigned to *political* reporters, not medical reporters, and the politicos naturally judge everything through a "can-this-pass" filter. Reporters, confronting a complicated subject, are generally afraid of asking questions when they think the answers must be obvious to everyone else. Politicians and interest-group spokesmen can therefore spin like tops, using statistics and scenarios that reporters don't know enough to challenge.

Even the "MacNeil-Lehrer NewsHour," which makes unusual efforts to air the full range of health care opinion, dramatizes the problems. In May health reporter Stuart Schear arranged a four-guest debate on single payer versus managed competition. One of the managed competition critics mysteriously dropped his opposition on the air, leaving only Steffie Woolhandler, a Harvard colleague of David Himmelstein, to make the Canadian case. At the end of the interview, MacNeil noted that Woolhandler was in the minority and then asked, "If this [managed competition] is the program that has political consensus and the other one that you advocate [single payer] is considered impossible politically at the moment, why are you then against the one that is viable and would produce a large amount of reform?"

Although Woolhandler rejected the assumption that managed competition would produce meaningful reform, MacNeil's question—designed as it may have been to elicit an interesting response—reinforced the impression that single payer was simply not feasible.

HEALTH SNARE

If most politicians dwell in fear of insurance industry enmity and political irrelevance, and if most reporters ingest that view without thinking, then where are we? Where can reporters and moderate and liberal politicians turn in the health care debate? Quick—to the Rolodex. How about the outside experts?

Unfortunately, the cultural imperatives that shut down political and journalistic inquiry are also at work in think tanks and universities. Experts fear being labeled as out of touch almost as much as the politicians and the press. Take Henry Aaron, the highly regarded senior economist at the Brookings Institution, whose 1991 book on health care, *Serious and Unstable Condition,* was widely noted in Washington. Aaron's book painstakingly reviews our troubled "condition," reports the experience of other industrial democracies, and then outlines a solution which in fact reflects principles applied abroad. But he devotes just one paragraph to Canada, and his proposed solution builds on private insurance. Intellectually honest, Aaron almost apologetically explains his surrender to presumed political constraint: "Although a wholly public plan probably could achieve some additional savings . . . [my plan] is predicated on the unwillingness of Congress to shift the bulk of currently private health care arrangements for most Americans." No one wants to be left out. Or perhaps it is more accurate to say that few policy intellectuals want to be marginalized.

To understand the pressures restricting scholarly research on the lessons of foreign experience, consider the following. In the 1970s, there was modest support for international study from the National Institutes of Health and other federal agencies. But in recent years NIH has provided very little financing for research on issues of health policy or foreign experience with universal health insurance. The result is that American experts are dependent on very few financial sources for broader work on health care reform, and most of those sources are not interested in cross-national research.

There are, of course, exceptions. The small Milbank Memorial Fund has provided financing for a limited number of discrete cross-national projects. So has the Pew Charitable Trust. The Commonwealth Fund did so briefly in the 1980s. But these are deviations from the pattern of

American foundations' health policy provincialism. The Robert Wood Johnson Foundation annually spends hundreds of millions of dollars on investigations of health care and financing, but little if any on cross-national work. The Johnson board has shied away from funding scholars outside the United States and is hesitant about American studies of foreign experience. The Ford Foundation, which has supported cross-national policy research in other fields, cedes health care to Johnson, Pew, and Rockefeller. The health interest of the Rockefeller Foundation has always been in medical sciences and, where cross-national and policy oriented, in the problems of the developing world.

Support for study of international health care is consequently stingy. When such studies *are* funded, grantors suggest or insist that overseas problems receive special emphasis. Indeed, some say there is a financial price to be paid if one goes too far beyond what is regarded as the conventional wisdom.

Consider again the case of David Himmelstein, the authority on the costs of bureaucracy in the American and Canadian health systems. His studies, conducted with Woolhandler, appear regularly in the *New England Journal of Medicine* and, though controversial, have been used by the General Accounting Office, journalists, and congressional committees to compare health systems. Yet their research has been done on a shoestring. The two doctors actually had to pool their academic salaries to pay research expenses. (And although the research is cited, it is not generally understood and runs into the usual journalistic he said/she said confusion.)

Private funding for research on single-payer systems is far more difficult to find than money for other kinds of health care research, Himmelstein says, unless you make clear that conclusions will be negative. "Research that may show the superiority of a single payer system is somewhere between difficult and impossible to fund." In 11 years, his sole funded project was "only indirectly related to single payer work." Himmelstein has been complaining of bias for years. One foundation vice president told him in confidence that his work would never be funded. "There is a person on our board," the foundation official said, "who will veto any proposal that would lead to the abolition of the health insurance industry. A specific piece of research that leads to the implication that the health insurance industry should be done away with is completely unfundable." Himmelstein looked around and saw that most of the foundation boards he was applying to had members connected to the insurance industry.

Of course, serious students of single-payer systems *can* be funded (full disclosure: both authors of this article have been); it's just harder, and that is important. Inside Washington, experts tend to play the game as it is played by the politicians and the press: focus on the possibilities of the moment. For that reason, both the Brookings Institution and the Urban Institute, the respectable left-of-center think tanks, now largely ignore single-payer plans. So there is an imbalance with important implications: reformers suck up to the "feasible," and the forces for the status quo spread the myths and exacerbate the problem.

The upshot of this relationship among journalists, politicians, and experts is confusion about Canada, not clarification of its enduring strengths and weaknesses. Sound-bite journalism—electronic and print, featuring snippets of contradictory claims—has obscured the fact that Canada, although recently suffering from recession, has managed to satisfy most of its citizens in ways we should marvel at and learn from, not dismiss.

Chapter 11
Hype and Hyperbole
in Health Reform

WITH JERRY MASHAW

To solve the problems of systems or even institutions, we need to look beyond the latest management fads and techniques.

We begin with a sad truth: "managed competition" is an oxymoron. A managed system is one under the control of actors who shape its operation by applying various managerial techniques. A competitive system is one that is up for grabs. Dispersed individuals, firms, and groups—all pursuing their own self-interests—interact to produce results that are not planned, perhaps not even desired, by anyone.

That the basic reform of medical care should be captured by a seemingly appealing and internally contradictory slogan is both disquieting and potentially instructive. Disquieting because it suggests that anyone who utters these words as a mantra-like solution to America's medical woes runs the grave risk of being considered an idiot or a fraud. Instructive because the juxtaposition of opposing ideas, bundled together into a new form, is the essence of managerial reform. Creative synthesis symbolizes but does not explain why management reform is a perpetual-

This chapter is a slightly revised version of "Rhetoric and Reality," *Health Management Quarterly*, Vol. 15, No. 4 (Winter 1993), pp. 21–24. Reprinted by permission.

Jerry Mashaw is the Gordon Bradford Tweedie Professor at the Yale Law School.

motion machine. The initiatives of one era necessarily give way to the enthusiasms of the next. Each management revolution launches itself with high hopes and inflated rhetoric, only to be abandoned later without regret.

This feature of American management need not cause despair. What we need instead is a more balanced view of the possibilities of managerial success and the basic determinants of managerial change. Better understanding of why the managerial world produces such cycles of enthusiasm followed by declarations of failure will probably never prevent the making of fortunes by distributing the managerial equivalent of snake oil. (Nor is it clear that a dose of snake oil from time to time is not good for the digestion.) Nevertheless, a little realism about what management can and cannot do for us might guard against swallowing the more noxious compounds offered by managerial innovators and help moderate our disappointment that good management has not rid us of all the world's evils.

Our readers, we assume, are familiar with the shifting sands of managerial theorizing. Whether in the public or private sector, American managers have developed, marketed, applied, and abandoned numerous approaches to common organizational problems. Two decades ago "management by objective" and "zero-based budgeting" were the rage. Managementspeak has shifted in recent years to hortatory labels such as "total quality management" and "integrated systems management." These are all slogans at one level. But they carry with them very different notions about the organizational goals to be emphasized, the internal relationships, the structure of authority that provides guidance, and the information or techniques necessary to make such reforms operate.

We have experimented with organizational models ranging from simple hierarchies with strict division of labor to cooperative teams. Ideal relationships between managers and employees have ranged from those emphasizing adversarial combat to others featuring bonding techniques reminiscent of summer camp or "two-a-day" football practice. And within these notions of organizational or systems design have arisen a dizzying array of techniques from "just in time" inventory management to statistical quality-assurance systems. In the medical field, the most recent technique is the much-heralded "outcomes measurement."

In one period, we think big is better. Good managers are supposed to be horizontally and vertically integrating firms and bureaus into ever-larger conglomerations of functions and product lines. The emphasis is on synergy, economies of scale, coordinated or unified central management, and the like. After a few years, however, we learn to think that small is beautiful. Divestiture, devolution, decentralization, focus, and specialization become the watchwords of right-thinking managers, public, private, and nonprofit.

It is tempting to suggest that management reform, like politics in Louisiana, is really part of the entertainment industry. Changing fads and fashions are simply necessary to stimulate our interest and keep us managing rather than going on vacation. But this is a view both too cynical and too simple. The endless cycling of fads, slogans, and techniques is the product of deeper forces that we ignore only at our peril. As we move into the new world of "managed competition"—or something that takes its place—we will do well to keep common sense in control. We need ideas that both explain the demand for managerial change and highlight the danger of believing that managerial techniques are the equivalent of *solutions* to the problems of our institutions.

The first simple truth is that institutional objectives are multiple, contradictory, and shifting. It would be surprising if a single managerial approach could cope effectively with differing objectives, or with changes over time in the ordering of priorities. Consider how one might answer the question, "What is the purpose of a hospital?" At different times, and often during the same period, we might at the very least give the following answers:

1. A hospital is designed to contain the spread of contagious diseases.
2. A hospital is a place that provides hygienic surroundings for otherwise dangerous activities.
3. A hospital is designed to economize on the cost of access to expensive technology.
4. A hospital provides respite from normal social roles that produce physical or emotional breakdown in patients.
5. Hospitals are intended to economize on information transmission and learning among professionals who have clinical responsibilities and a need for repeated clinical encounters to validate their procedures.
6. Hospitals are designed to centralize health-related activities sufficiently to achieve economies of scale in the pursuit of separable medical care tasks.
7. Hospitals provide symbolic reassurance that we are devoting social effort to the health of individuals in a culture that has a considerable faith in technological remedies.

8. Hospitals are institutions designed to improve a population's health.

The list could go on and on. Even in this truncated version the hospital has social, medical, health, professional, economic, and educational missions. But not all of these purposes are attainable through the same structures of internal authority, using the same informational technologies, or operating on the same time scales.

Moreover, the purposes give rise to starkly different images of successful operation. An emphasis on purpose 4, for example, would imply a very relaxed approach to patient length of stay, whereas an emphasis on purpose 3 or purpose 6 might view longer hospital stays as evidence of managerial failure. An emphasis on purpose 5 suggests a team approach to management with authority centralized in professionals, whereas an emphasis on purpose 3 might well encourage a hierarchical organization with the extensive use of bureaucratic authority. Note also that while purposes 1 through 7 imply allocations of authority somewhere *within* the hospital as an institution, purpose 8 might be thought to call for a much broader authority structure, including outside stakeholders with the power to define and redefine the institution's primary mission.

The lesson here is obvious. Medical institutions such as hospitals have multiple tasks that require different organizational structures and techniques—in short, different managerial approaches. The issue of good management is not what slogan the hospital administrator has decided to emblazon across the employees' T-shirts or scrub suits. Instead, it is how well the managerial approach balances the differentiated demands of the institution's multiple purposes. We would not belabor this basic point but for the overwhelming evidence that it is often forgotten. When some Tom Peters clone next says to health care managers that to have multiple objectives, or even two objectives, is to have no objectives, he should be taken out and thrown—not merely asked to jump—into the nearest lake.

Consider a second simple truth about managerial technique that is intimately related to the existence of multiple objectives: every upside has a downside. As we move willy-nilly into the world of "managed care," if not managed competition, we must reflect on what may be lost as well as gained. Whether the technique is preapproval for specialist care or hospitalization, or movement to a staff-model HMO for providing services, managed care concentrates on eliminating unnecessary physician-patient encounters, diagnostic procedures, surgical interventions, and pharmaceutical prescriptions. The bureaucratic routines necessary for these activities may well control costs (some better than others, some not at all), but the potential loss of patient and physician autonomy, control over quality, and profit-driven innovation may be significant. A range of different managerial techniques, organizations, and institutions will be required if these values are not to be sacrificed to the god of Cost Containment. Moreover, the techniques implied by managed care (hierarchy, routinized information collection, and the like) are not the same techniques that will facilitate innovation, patient control, or professional satisfaction. Intoning "TQM" (Total Quality Management) or "integrated systems management" will not eliminate the stress that is built into serving different purposes and clienteles having multiple aims. Good management entails the use of varied means to balance the "goods" and "bads" of each approach.

Third, we think it is important to recognize that the internal and external environments of organizations are different. Changes in management form and technique usually require changes in the internal structures and procedures of organizations. Often, however, these changes are driven by the necessity to respond to the external environment. When the external political environment in 1965, for example, signaled the medical care industry that its major goal should be elimination of the insecurity of health care for the aged, the managerial response was sensible and straightforward: organize the system to attract physicians into it by paying their reasonable and customary charges, and impose few or no restraints on their individual autonomy or form of medical practice. In the deficit politics of the 1970s, 1980s, and 1990s, the Health Care Financing Administration's managerial task has been rather different. Devolution of choice—of both treatments and price—to physicians has been replaced by ever-more-centralized means of overseeing physicians' choices and regulating their rates. The same is true of hospitals. Managerial issues that were thought to be internal to the institution have now come under substantial control by outside stakeholders. In the process, the internal organization of medical care institutions and medical practices has shifted to cope with these external demands.

Changes in the external environment of an institution or system may be the key determinants of managerial reform. From an internal perspective, a hospital administrator might well want to manage an institution primarily through devolution of authority to teams of physicians and their assistants, whose focus is on patient care and quality improvement. As a realist in a world of constrained resources, the hospital administrator may instead be required to emphasize the hierarchical authority of the financial vice president and exalt the status of the people who do wallet biopsies and labor negotiations.

Finally, we want to emphasize a deep ambivalence in managerial theory concerning the efficacy of technological versus cultural solutions to managerial problems. Ever since "Taylorism" provoked a reaction based on that particular model's desire to treat people and machines as interchangeable, management theorists have oscillated between recommendations based on structures, processes, and technologies and those based on learning, motivation, and culture. We cannot decide which managerial strategy to believe in, because both work some of the time but not all of the time.

The same will be true in the reorganization of America's health care system. It is hard to believe that a cultural approach will be attractive from a standpoint of cost containment. Managed care is about information systems, statistical testing, and scientifically determining what works or what is cost effective. On the other hand, if we move to a world of HMOs we are likely to want to retain the cultural vision of Marcus Welby—doctor, counselor, and friend. If so, we will want some internal structures that emphasize professional autonomy, team effort, group responsibility for care, and patient involvement in an overall culture of "wellness." Our managerial arrangements will to some degree work at cross-purposes—the technocracy of cost containment confronting the professional culture of patient care. The trick of good management will be to balance these perspectives in ways that cope with our conflicting purposes and inconsistent desires.

This brings us to our final point. Management, in health care as elsewhere, is not a *solution* to inevitable systemic stresses. It is a means of coping with and sometimes improving situations that are only marginally tractable. Such a modest vision of management has much to teach politicians and policymakers and anyone else engaged in designing or reforming complex systems. Management cannot teach other fields that lesson, however, until it gives up the quasi-religious adoption of one management slogan or technique after another as "the solution" to getting management right. There is no best management theory, technique, or slogan. But in particular contexts, some *are* better than others.

Part III

Comparative Perspectives

Chapter 12
Patterns of Fact and Fiction in
Use of the Canadian Experience

As of this writing (June 1993), the preoccupation of the United States with health care reform hardly seems to involve Canada. During his 1992 campaign, President Clinton did repeatedly cite the superior experience of other industrial democracies, including Canada, in controlling health costs. But he seldom embraced Canada's Medicare as a model of national health insurance. Indeed, one noticed his innocent repetition of some of the myths which the American Medical Association (AMA) and the Health Insurance Association of America (HIAA) have, along with others, relentlessly disseminated during the most recent period of political interest in Canada (roughly from 1989 to early 1992). Canada has played a crucial if not-well-understood role in American debates over health care since the late 1960s and even today has an influence that is all too easy to overlook now that the nation's media are preoccupied with understanding the newest slogan for reform, "managed competition."[1]

The history of U.S. interest in Canadian public health insurance is mostly a story of episodes of public discussion and interest (1970–1974,

Reprinted by permission from the *American Review of Canadian Studies*, Vol. 23, No. 1 (Spring 1993), pp. 47–64. This article is an updated and expanded version of a piece in the December 1991 issue of *Current History*. Copyright © 1991, Current History, Inc. Used by permission.

1989–1992) punctuated by longer periods of inattention. Before the 1970s, very few health policy analysts in the United States knew much about Canadian experience or paid much attention to it. Among the exceptions were scholars like Cecil Sheps and Sam Wolfe, Canadians who participated in Canada's reforms during the postwar period, emigrated to the United States, and continued to write about Canadian experience and its relevance to the United States. But the number was small, as I learned when I turned to North American comparative studies in the late 1960s.

As we shall see, that was not to remain true in the 1970s. Early in the decade, Senator Edward M. Kennedy (D., Mass.) was the most prominent example of the many politicians who traveled north to marvel at Canada's relative success and celebrated its lessons upon return. In 1973 and 1974, national health insurance was firmly on the American political agenda, and the Kennedy-Corman plan of that period owed much to the Canadian model. The 1975 book *National Health Insurance: Can We Learn from Canada?* was widely read in academic and policy circles, and Canadian scholars such as Robert Evans of the University of British Columbia were regular participants in seminars and conferences south of their border.[2]

Canada's Medicare faded from public view in parallel with the fading of national health insurance from the U.S. national agenda. It is easy to forget that Jimmy Carter ran for president partly on the promise to enact national health insurance, and there was enough interest in the late 1970s to warrant a steady flow of papers and occasional books. But the Reagan years were tough ones for North American comparativists. The frustration with stagflation and the same neoconservative forces that brought Prime Minister Brian Mulroney to Canada had their effect. The crises of the welfare state and the call for deregulation and the retrenchment of the state brought procompetitive arguments to the fore.[3] It took until 1989 for a serious interest in Canadian Medicare to reappear. And then it emerged in a familiar manic-depressive cycle of initial excitement, manic coverage, and depressive reaction.

The precipitants of excitement are easy enough to identify. In 1989 Lee Iacocca, the head of Chrysler, and his board member and former Carter cabinet officer, Joseph Califano, published admiring editorials in the *New York Times*. Though nothing new was being said, new figures were arguing that Canada's form of national health insurance combined broader coverage and less cost than in the United States and, furthermore, that our persistent medical inflation was a serious problem for the competitiveness of U.S. corporations. What followed was a torrent of attention—from squads of Congresspeople visiting Montreal, Toronto, and Vancouver to numerous newspaper features, from public television's 1990 documentary *Borderline Medicine* to the persistently favorable reviews of Canadian experience by a new medical group, Physicians for a National Health Plan (PNHP). All three television networks did specials on Canada's experience with Medicare, and for a time Canadian experts were inundated with requests for interviews, information, and expertise. Had the 1992 election been held in 1990, Canada would have figured prominently in it.

The forces of reaction, however, had ample time to develop. Led by the AMA initially, the critics of Canada's "socialized medicine" used the full arsenal of propagandistic techniques to question both Canada's performance and its relevance to the United States.[4] The HIAA came to take the lead role here, shamelessly blasting a favorable report by the Government Accounting Office in 1991 as "partisan." The public paid less attention to this than the politicians, overwhelmingly stating their approval of the Canadian program pollsters described to them. But the growth of a vigorous pro- and anti-Canada lobby took its toll on risk-averse presidential candidates.

All of this was played out in dramatic form during the Democratic primaries of 1992. Senator Bob Kerrey, an admirer of Canadian health insurance, advanced a plan similar to Medicare, but increasingly distanced himself from explicit citation of the model. He came to talk, as did others, of the need for an "American solution" for an "American problem," hoping to avoid the knee-jerk nativism that rises close to the surface of American public life whenever it is claimed that another nation has something to teach us. And with that attitude came additional commentary that Canada, after all, was really quite different from the United States.[5]

The mixture of superficial programmatic and cultural analysis has taken its toll. Bill Clinton heard more about Canada's troubles and its cultural distinctiveness than he did about how Canada's comparative success reflected policies and structures that international experience validated as cross-national lessons. In this he was not helped by Canadians who, in an understandable concern for differentiating themselves from the United States and fearing for the fate of national health insurance under free trade, kept repeating the claim that Canada was so different from the United States as was France or Germany. Never was so much North American bunk disseminated so widely, despite the warnings of comparativists like Keith Banting, Morris Barer, Uwe Reinhardt, or Humphrey Taylor.[6]

The painful pressures of recession have now made health care reform a leading issue in the United States and, at the same time, have highlighted Canada's current strains. The discussion in the United States reflects this twin reality, and the result is a debate that seldom mentions anything but Canada's troubles. In February 1992, President Bush still felt it necessary to attack Canada's experience as largely a "failure" and, in any event, irrelevant. (That caused a minor stir in Canada, with three provincial premiers on television the next morning to denounce the president's ignorance of Canadian reality.) But by December the vice president of the HIAA complacently stated on cable television that the "American people are not ready for a Canadian-style government solution." And, as the *New York Times* continues to celebrate "managed competition," its editorial writer persistently dismisses the "bureaucratic" solution of Canada. Voices of reason persist, most prominently the Consumer's Union (which published in the summer of 1992 an excellent guide to national health insurance that portrayed Canada as a troubled but undeniable model); Congressman Jim McDermott, former Congressman Marty Russo, and Senator Paul Wellstone; Kathy Hurwitt of Citizen Action; as well as the writings of PNHP analysts Steffie Woolhandler, David Himmelstein, and Thomas Bodenheimer. But the undeniable fact is that Canada's Medicare is not at the moment a leading contender for the reform soul of President Clinton.

Does that mean Canadian experience has been rendered useless, or its impact reduced to the musings of scholars? I think not, but explaining why is not simple. Consider that in 1991 journalists assumed that play-or-pay plans were likely to emerge from the play of American politics, and none of them even mentioned the category of a "global budget." At this writing, most journalists are commenting on the possibility of "managed competition within the context of a global budget," repeating the very words President Clinton used in the last weeks of his campaign. The principles announced by the presidential transition team on health include universality, global budget limits, state involvement, comprehensive benefits, and managed care. All but the last reflect Canadian principles! And the pairing of global budgets and universality reflects the seeping into the U.S. reform mind of precisely the key elements analysts of Canadian experience have been emphasizing for two decades. It is true that the decreased appeal (to politicians) of the single-payer model has discouraged many citizen activists groups who know the American public is well disposed to Canada's experience and anxious to rid us of the wasteful administrative expense of 1,500 private insurers. Still, it would be a great mistake to overlook the impact that

Canadian experience has had or to believe that the labels used to refer to a reform plan fully illuminate its features or the forces that produced them.

GROWING INTEREST IN CHANGE: 1989–1991

If there is any part of American life that is regularly criticized as unaffordable, unfair, and uncontrollable, it is medical care. The claim that American medicine is "in crisis" is of course not new—both Senator Kennedy and President Nixon agreed on that in 1971. What is new is the extension of alarm to American business leaders, who are seriously worried about skyrocketing health insurance premiums and whose complaints have transformed the media's coverage of American medicine.

One sign of this transformed discussion is the unexpected prominence of Canada's health care system in American debates over what can and should be done about the medical care "crisis" in the United States. Between 1989 and 1991 especially, commissions and commentators took up the topic of serious reform in American medical care with vigor. Not only did Iacocca and Califano write widely cited pieces criticizing American medical practices and lauding Canada's national health insurance program, but the PNHP published its recommendation of a "Canadian-style" plan in the *New England Journal of Medicine*.[7]

Whatever the catalyst, the Canadian model gained popularity with media commentators, surprising Canadians so accustomed to American neglect. Congressional committees began to ask Canadian experts to testify, and political organizations sent parades of representatives to Canada on crash study tours. But the most striking evidence of the seriousness with which American commentators have taken the Canadian model were the attacks on it by the American Medical Association.

Under the seemingly innocently titled "Public Alert Program," the AMA committed $2.5 million in 1989 to "telling millions of Americans the facts about the Canadian health-care system." In a campaign reminiscent of its 1984 attack on President Harry Truman's proposed national health insurance scheme, the AMA began to place advertisements in the major media and to supply background materials for a blitz of editorials, opinion pieces, and reports about Canada.

Why should the AMA have been so concerned about the Canadian example of national health insurance? Why, in turn, should the Health Insurance Association of America have devoted expensive staff energy to producing what amounts to a book asserting that no matter how appealing the Canadian model is, it would be neither politically accept-

able nor practical to implement?[8] The answer is not terribly complicated. Business, labor, and popular discontent with American medicine
has crystallized. There is widespread political interest in substantial
change, and the Canadian example has been used widely enough for
criticism to warrant counterattack from those with the greatest stake in
the status quo.

Contrary to the message of the AMA and the HIAA, the Canadian
system not only works reasonably well—it pays for universal access to
ordinary medical care, maintains a generally high level of quality, is
administratively efficient, and restrains the growth of health care costs
far more effectively than any of the myriad cost containment schemes
tried in the United States—but is as adaptable to American circumstances as one could imagine a foreign model to be.

CAN THE UNITED STATES LEARN FROM ABROAD?

Canada, France, and Germany provide their citizens with universal health insurance coverage at a cost of between 8 and 9.5 percent
of GNP. Britain, Japan, and Australia provide it for between 6 and 8
percent of GNP. The United States, as is so often noted, spends more
than 12 percent of GNP on health care—more than any other country—
and yet ranks below all the members of the Organization for European
Cooperation and Development in terms of infant mortality and life
expectancy. For all the money spent, there are still some 37 million
Americans without health insurance and an undetermined number who
have inadequate insurance. The United States is obviously doing something wrong.

When other countries achieve what the United States says it would
like to attain, it makes good sense to look abroad. But for Americans
there are particularly revealing difficulties in looking abroad for lessons—whether in government or commerce. The American public is
somewhat skittish about America's uniqueness, educated to believe in
the special mission and character of this "city on a hill." Cross-national
comparisons can easily arouse xenophobia, with defenders of the status
quo ever ready to invoke the claim that "America is just different."

Three dangers complicate the politics of American-Canadian health
care policy arguments. First is the widespread incidence of well-
financed distortion, the mythmaking exemplified by the AMA campaign.
Second is the mistaken notion that if there is any way in which two
nations differ, they are not "comparable." (There are some hilarious
examples of this fallacy of comparative difference in the recent media

attention to Canada. One claim of Canada's irrelevance to the United States, written by a "surgeon from White Plains" for the opinion page of the *New York Times*,[9] noted the fact that 90 percent of Canada's population lives within 100 miles of the American border.)

Less hilarious but more important working illustrations of the fallacy of comparative difference show up regularly in the comments of American health care policy analysts. For instance, Alain Enthoven, a Stanford University economist who has closely examined American medical reform, frankly admits Canada's superior performance but challenges its relevance. In a debate in the summer of 1990 about what to do about America's medical "mess," Enthoven argued against wasting any more time talking about Canada. Canadian culture and politics are so different, he alleged, that a serious attempt to borrow from their undeniably good experience was "off the radar screen of American possibility."[10]

The assertion that Canada's experience is not relevant is supported by sociologist Seymour Martin Lipset, a thoughtful and nuanced commentator on North American similarities and differences.[11] According to Lipset, Canadians respect government far more than Americans do, a contention buttressed by the difference between the Canadian founding document and the American Declaration of Independence. According to their charter, Canadians are committed to "peace, order, and good government," while Americans look to the individualistic "pursuit of happiness."

Never has so much been claimed with so little evidence; serious comparative research on public opinion shows no fundamental difference between the North American publics—a somewhat wider range on the Canadian left to be sure, but a distribution that leads most comparativists to group the United States and Canada together as similar liberal democracies in their creeds.

Canada's path to and experience with national health insurance provides American policymakers with a perfect opportunity for cross-national learning. The United States shares with Canada a common language and political roots, a comparably diverse population with a similar distribution of living standards, increasingly integrated economies, and a tradition of fractious but constitutional federalism that makes political disputes similar though obviously not identical. Moreover, until Canada consolidated its national health insurance in 1971, the patterns and styles of medical care in both countries were nearly identical. (Indeed, Canadian regulators used the United States Joint Commission on Hospital Accreditation to judge their hospitals' acceptability until well after World War II.)

Three questions emerge in examining the Canadian Health care experience. The first is whether Canada's medical care system is truly exemplary and worth importing. The second is whether a Canadian-style program is politically feasible in the United States. And third, even if desirable as a model and politically acceptable, can Canadian national health insurance be adapted to American circumstances?

CANADA'S EXEMPLARY PERFORMANCE

The basic outline of Canada's national health insurance is clear. The federal government conditionally promises each province that it will prepay roughly 40 percent of the costs of all necessary medical care. The federal grant is available so long as the province's health insurance program is universal (covering all citizens), comprehensive (covering all conventional hospital and medical care), accessible (no limits on services and no extra charges to patients), portable (each province recognizes the others' coverage), and publicly administered (under control of a public, nonprofit organization). All ten provinces maintain health insurance plans satisfying these criteria. The provincial ministry of health is the only payer in each province. There are no complex eligibility tests or complicated definitions of insured services. Administrative costs, as a consequence, are negligible by American standards.

The practical dynamics of Canada's program are also simple, at least in outline. Annual negotiations between provincial governments and the providers of care determine the hospital budgets and the level of physicians' fees. As in the United States, most hospitals are nonprofit community institutions and physicians practice (under fee-for-service payment) in diverse individual and group settings. Patients choose their own doctors; doctors bill the province; and hospitals work from global budgets, not itemized billings. Disagreements over insurance claims, gaps in coverage, and bureaucratic incomprehensibility are, for practical purposes, nonexistent. Canadian patients and providers never have to file multiple claims to different insurers. (American Medicare beneficiaries might well have to file claims with three or more insurers, and a physician or hospital treating Medicaid patients might have to wait six months or more for payment.)

Most of the negative effects predicted by economic theory and Canadian doctors—worrisome physician flight, rationing of lifesaving care, long queues, and technological obsolescence—have not emerged. There is, and has always been, some movement of highly trained, highly prized

Table 12.1
Physicians per 100,000 people, United States and Canada

Year	United States	Canada
1965	155	130
1970	159	146
1975	178	172
1980	201	184
1985	224	206
1987	234	216

Source: Organization for Economic Cooperation and Development, *Health Care Systems in Transition: The Search For Efficiency.* Paris: OECD, 1990, Tables 27 and 61.

personnel from Canada to the United States. Physicians are no exception. But this trend was not greatly affected by Canadian national health insurance, and the numbers have always been small, not enough to offset a steady increase in the number of practicing physicians. As Table 12.1 shows, Canada's physician population ratio has been, and remains, comparable to that of the United States.

At the outset, the existing physician fee schedules of provincial medical associations were accepted by the provincial governments, although in most provinces payments were initially set somewhat below 100 percent to reflect the elimination of a doctor's risk of unpaid debts. Since that time, changes in the fee schedules have been negotiated by provincial medical associations and ministries of health. The typical process of setting fees is one of extended negotiation, not unilateral imposition. Physicians were the highest-paid professionals in Canada before the introduction of universal medical insurance; they still are.

Canada does ration medical care. So does the United States and every other country in the world. What counts is not the presence of rationing (or allocation) but the basis for and the extent of restricted access to health care. The United States continues to ration by the ability to pay—a process largely determined by race, class, and employment circumstances. Access to care and the quality of care vary enormously, and many in the United States—particularly the poor or the poorly insured—experience long waiting lists and substandard facilities, if they receive care at all. By contrast, Canada and most other developed countries try to provide a more uniform standard of care to

Table 12.2
Comparative availability of selected medical technologies, United States and Canada (units per million people)

Medical technology	U.S.	Canada	Ratio U.S. to Canada
Open-heart surgery	3.26	1.23	2.7:1
Cardiac catheterization	5.06	1.50	3.4:1
Organ transplantation	1.31	1.08	1.2:1
Radiation therapy	3.97	0.54	7.4:1
Extracorporeal shock wave lithoscopy	0.94	0.16 (1988)	5.9:1
Magnetic resonance imaging	3.69	0.46	8.0:1

Note: United States data are for 1987, Canada for 1989, except where indicated.
Source: D. A. Rublee, "Medical Technology in Canada and the U.S.," *Health Affairs* 1989 (Fall):180. Reprinted by permission.

the entire population. Medical care is allocated largely on the basis of relative medical need, which is determined by physician judgment, not by insurance status, bureaucratic rules, or arbitrary age limits.

At certain times and in some places, substantial waiting lists for selected surgical and diagnostic procedures occur. Nevertheless, the overall rates of hospital use per capita are considerably higher in Canada than in the United States. Most patients are cared for in a timely manner, and long waiting lists reflect managerial problems more than chronic shortages of facilities. Emergency care is available immediately to everyone.

There is no question that some expensive, high-technology items are not as available in Canada as they are in the United States. Canada has a full range of high-technology facilities, but in considerably less abundance and with little competition for market share. Expensive capital equipment is first approved only for highly specialized centers, and subsequent diffusion is closely controlled by provincial ministries of health. This control results in lower rates of use for some technologies in Canada—cardiac surgery, magnetic resonance imaging, lithoscopy, and so on (see Table 12.2). This is not necessarily a bad thing. Throughout North America there is concern about the appropriate use of expensive new procedures. Inappropriate use is both financially costly and medically dangerous to patients.

The quality of a nation's health care is never simple to measure. Many critics view the slower diffusion and limited use of some new technologies in Canada as evidence of lower-quality care. If quality is defined as more high-technology services regardless of relative effectiveness, then the United States certainly offers higher-quality medical care. If, however, quality is defined by health results rather than by the use of high technology, then there is no evidence of a Canadian disadvantage. If life expectancy and infant mortality measure the quality of a health care system, Canada has a definite advantage. And if consumer satisfaction is a critical component of quality, then both polls and political behavior put Canadian national health insurance well in the lead.

The generally high levels of Canadian satisfaction suggest the importance of the way health care quality is distributed. When quality is defined as the best technologies and facilities available to the most privileged members of a population, rather than as the facilities available to the average individual, American medical care ranks among the best in the world. But major aspects of American medical care—the limited extent of immunization, the large number of pregnant women without regular medical attention, and the risk of bankruptcy from illness—would be considered intolerable in other comparably wealthy countries. Canada has fewer centers of technological excellence, but the average level of care is, by any definition, at least equal to that in the United States.

ADAPTING CANADA'S HEALTH CARE SYSTEM

What would make the Canadian option not only more attractive to the American electorate, but also easier to implement in the American context? Part of the answer lies in distinguishing the necessary from the incidental elements of the Canadian success story. The Canadian program combines three features that have made its cost, access, and quality acceptable over nearly twenty years of full-scale operation.

One of the features is universality of coverage. All Canadians are insured on the "same terms and conditions." This universality has made it politically impossible in Canada to deal with cost pressures by stealth or to permit end runs around the controls. Second, there is a clear center of financial responsibility in Canada: a ministry of health or its equivalent in each province. Financing medical care under concentrated rather than fragmented auspices is crucial to the third component of Canada's system: unambiguous political accountability for the cost and quality of and access to Canadian medical care. These three features—

universal access, a responsible financing agency, and accountable political leaders—explain why Canada's performance has been superior
to that of the United States.

What do these features of the Canadian model mean for possible
American adaptations? What sorts of changes could be made without
losing what has been necessary for Canada's relatively successful experience with national health insurance?

Canada's universalism is strong in two ways. Every Canadian is
literally on the same provincial health insurance plan as his or her
neighbor—the equivalent of every Californian belonging to one Blue
Cross/Blue Shield plan. Furthermore, Canadians have the same coverage under their provincial plan: "equal terms and conditions," not varied
options. In the health sphere, Canada is probably more egalitarian than
any other comparable industrial democracy. Private insurers are forbid-
den by law to sell supplementary coverage for publicly insured services.
And to maintain the "equal terms" of access, Canadian doctors since
1984 have for all practical purposes been prevented from charging patients anything above the government's fee schedule.

Not all of these Canadian features are necessary for an acceptable
form of universal health insurance. Canada did not start with such a
firmly egalitarian version. The Hall Commission of 1964 to 1966, the
royal commission that justified extending government hospital insurance
to medical care, defined universal coverage as no less than 95 percent
of the citizens in each province. While desirable on egalitarian grounds,
literal universality has not been a necessary feature of Canada's success.
American reformers need not insist on Canada's strong contemporary
form of universal enrollment.

"Uniform" conditions would also be less compelling than in Canada.
For Americans to be in the same boat does not necessarily require that
the boat's cabins all be the same size or have the same view. What is
essential is that the health insurance boat include most Americans on
roughly comparable terms.

It is on the issue of the terms of benefits and the constraints on
"supplementation" that the most acrimonious disputes are likely to
break out. Could the United States (or a state) forgo the Canadian ban
on supplementary health insurance for services covered under a universal plan without losing financial control? Would it be unacceptable
to permit physicians (or other medical professionals paid under fee-for-
service arrangements) to charge their patients more than the agreed-on
schedule of fees?

The answer here is ambiguous. On the first point, Canada has never experimented. But other nations with acceptable national health insurance programs have supplementary insurance that coexists with public coverage. As for charges that are above negotiated rates ("extra billing" or "balance billing" in the jargon of health economics), the answer is clearer. The ability to contain medical costs depends on establishing firm limits; extra billing violates those limits and reintroduces barriers to access that universal health insurance is meant to lower. No successful national health insurance program has permitted this practice for long; Canada found over time that balance billing became a serious problem in many communities, threatening both the uniformity of treatment and the access to treatment itself. Both supplementary insurance and extra billing, when widespread, threaten equitable cost control.

FINANCING NATIONAL HEALTH CARE

Whether Canada's concentration of finance in provincial ministries of health has been crucial to its successful control of medical care costs is the second issue to evaluate. Is the location of responsibility at the provincial as opposed to federal level vital? The other key question is whether Canada's public financing and direct governmental administration are required for political accountability: an identifiable budget accounts for a jurisdiction's overall health expenditure.

The cross-national evidence on the first question suggests that it is the concentration of financial responsibility, not its precise location, that is crucial to countervailing inflationary health care cost pressures. Canada, by constitutional requirement, had no choice but to use provincial governments to administer health insurance. Great Britain, by contrast, concentrates financial responsibility in the national ministry of health, and Sweden does so in each of its county councils. The lesson for the United States is that there are options.

The second, more difficult question concerns the direct accountability of the processes by which health care funds are raised and spent. Public financing makes Canadian outlays for health highly visible. At the same time, Canadian provinces could, and some did, use preexisting health insurance companies as political buffers between physicians and the government. In the mid-1960s, Ontario used these intermediaries to manage the flow of funds and the processing of claims. Such a buffer seemed important then as a concession to the deep hostility many Canadian doctors felt regarding government medical insurance. In fact, the Canadian provinces that used financial intermediaries at the outset abandoned them after a few years. They made administration complicated and more expensive, and once their role in moderating conflict was no longer necessary, they seemed useless (except to the insurance companies).

One can certainly imagine the use of such intermediaries in the United States. This, after all, has been the pattern with American Medicare since 1965—an arrangement that draws on private expertise and "economizes" on the number of public employees. Canadians found such indirect management cumbersome and more expensive to manage than direct administration. But contracting out financial tasks is certainly, on the Canadian evidence, compatible with political accountability.

In the United States of the 1990s, however, the crucial political problem facing national health insurance advocates is the public's hostility toward increased taxes. Can one imagine Canadian-style government health insurance working without direct public finance? In other words, what would be lost if, for example, state regulatory authorities set the terms of medical care financing, negotiated with hospitals and physicians, and required that employers finance health insurance directly or pay into a state fund a fixed amount per employee? However the point is phrased, the question remains the same: is it possible to have the right level of countervailing power without the fusion of taxing and negotiating responsibility?

The answer to that question is far from obvious. In some European countries—Germany in particular—national and state governments have played a powerful regulatory role without Canada's single-payer feature. The German government constrains the negotiations among physicians, hospitals, and the thousands of sickness funds without channeling social insurance financing through conventional public tax accounts. It sets the rules by which the parties operate, and each of the sickness funds faces the full financial consequences of its members' medical care. There is both financial accountability and complicated administration in the German example. The United States should notice that it does not have the German history of lifelong involvement with one health insurance institution.

What this suggests is that the degree of responsibility for health financing—and the clarity about where that accountability lies—is not solely determined by the details of public finance. There are forms of mandated health insurance, which finances care on terms negotiated by public officials, that might closely resemble in practice the publicly financed, compulsory health insurance program found in Canada.

It is certainly possible to imagine mandated universal health insur-

ance—with workable regulations drawn from German experience—
working tolerably well in the United States. Such arrangements could
address the problems of inflation, inadequate coverage, and political
accountability, but less effectively than a system modeled after Canada's. The United States should be under no illusion here; there are
choices available, with different trade-offs among acceptability, effectiveness, and administrative complexity. What the United States has at
the moment is a vicious circle of trouble; a system like Canada's is
possible, but a less direct program would be an improvement.

This sort of reasoning led some policy analysts to suggest adapting
the Canadian model along the lines suggested earlier. Their proposal
treats the state health department as the negotiating agent of universal
health insurance, insurance made universal by the accretion of mandated coverage for workers and their families, Medicare for those over
age 65 and the disabled, Medicaid for the poor, and a new insurance
plan for those not in these categories. No one starting from a blank
slate would seek this rather complicated version of universal coverage
through aggregation, clear public responsibility for costs, and decentralized administration. But, as a third choice, it should be tolerable.[12]

THE CASE FOR THE CANADIAN MODEL

In the early 1970s, American experts paid considerable attention
to Canada's recently completed program of national health insurance.
That scrutiny was part of the substantial interest in an American form
of universal health insurance. When the realities of stagflation in the
1970s and early 1980s removed national health insurance from the American political agenda, the lessons of Canada's experience were put aside,
hardly noticed except by specialists in health policy. The reawakening
of American interest in Canada comes without anything like a widely
shared American appreciation of how Canadian health insurance works
in practice.

The result of the disparity between interest and knowledge is a very
uneven discussion of what the United States can and cannot learn from
its neighbor to the north, let alone what adaptations to American circumstances a conscious effort to borrow from Canada's example would
entail. Instead, the discussion of Canadian health insurance resembles
a shouting match: enthusiasts point to evidence about citizen satisfaction and relatively low expenditures per capita, and detractors argue
either that Canada is too different for the United States to take seriously

as a model or that the model itself is terrible because it creates long lines, causes doctors to emigrate, and disappoints patients.

If there is any country from which the United States can learn, it is Canada. Having had similar medical care arrangements for most of the twentieth century, Canada and the United States have conducted over the past 20 years a fateful experiment in forms of medical finance. It is two decades and hundreds of billions of dollars too late to contend that the United States should have acted on Canadian lessons in the early 1970s. That option simply was not politically available in the economic aftermath of the first oil crisis in 1973. But that does not mean, in the 1990s and beyond that Americans cannot learn from Canada's example.

The central lesson of the Canadian experiment is that the balance among cost, quality, and access is relatively easy to evaluate. What Canada illustrates clearly is that a sensibly organized national health insurance system can work in a political community like that in the United States; that universal coverage, coherent financial responsibility, and clear political accountability are the central ingredients of success; and that a population accustomed to the same standard of medical care as the United States can take pride in what in essence are ten provincial Blue Cross/Blue Shield plans with comprehensive benefits to which everyone belongs as a matter of right. If that were thoroughly understood, the problems of adapting the Canadian model to America would seem less daunting.

Chapter 13
Japan—A Sobering Lesson

Since the spring of 1989, there has been a new twist to the crisis-talk about American medicine. The media have increasingly turned their attention to foreign experience, often admiringly so. In 1989, there was a flurry of interest in Canada's national health insurance following Lee Iaccoca's newspaper editorial claiming that we should, if we could, use Canada's Medicare as a model. In 1990, Germany became the medical example of the year, prompting a flurry of emergency visits by medical journalists and policy statesmen.

The skeptic might rightly ask, what really can we learn from abroad? That, of course, depends on what we are looking for: a model health insurance program, generalizations about successful cost containment, or predictions of developments from nations roughly similar to ours. Whatever the goal, at some point attention will surely turn toward Japan, though few American commentators have yet looked in that direction.[1]

If we are doing poorly with medical care, Japan, one might well assume, does it better. Right? After all, what doesn't Japan do better

Reprinted by permission from *Health Management Quarterly*, Vol. 14, No. 3 (Third Quarter 1992), pp. 10–14. Copyright © 1992 The Baxter Foundation. The author warmly acknowledges the research and editing assistance of M. Barr, R. Gribbon, C. Grobler, and S. Schwartz.

Deaths per 1,000 live births

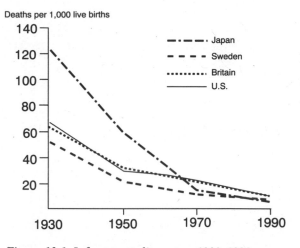

Figure 13.1 Infant mortality rates, 1930–1990.
Source: *United Nations Demographic Year-
book,* 1951, 1960, 1972, 1990.

than the United States—other than football, rock music, and the pursuit
of leisure? Well, delivering excellent medical care that satisfies patients
and payers turns out not to be an example of Japanese superiority.
Quite the contrary: while Japan is admirably healthy, the quality of its
medical system is decided mixed.

That Japan's health indices are excellent cannot be disputed. Its
infant mortality rate is half that of the United States. From a base of
124 infant deaths per thousand in 1930, the rate fell to 12 in 1970 and
halved again to the present rate of 5 deaths per thousand. During that
same period, life expectancy at birth increased from 45 years to 76 for
Japanese males and from 47 to 81 for Japanese females.[2] These improvements are consistent with trends toward increased longevity and reduced infant deaths throughout the developed world, but Japan has
accomplished them better than others—and more recently. Indeed, Japan's record on these gross measures of health is now the best in the
world, surpassing Sweden's in the last few years. This leap to the top
of the world tables was hardly foreordained; Japan's starting point in
the postwar period was shockingly low (Figure 13.1).

Sounds wonderful. But few experts believe that the quality of Japan's
surgical and medical teams is the main explanation for the population's
good health. Japanese medicine is full of trouble spots: lavish—perhaps
questionable—use of prescription drugs, small hospitals that would
strike most Americans as cottage institutions, unevenly trained physi-

cians for whom income and quality are practically inversely related, and much more. Japan's hospitals and clinics compete fiercely for patients, and the competition, according to most commentators, does not make for good medical care. Indeed, as Naoki Ikegami of Keio University Medical School in Tokyo has characterized Japanese medical patterns, one sees few grounds for imitation:

> Much of the power and prestige is concentrated in the professors of medical schools. . . . Most hospitals recruit physicians through the professors' informal patronage and recommendations without formal appraisal. Because of this, more objective postgraduate qualifications to evaluate individual physicians have not developed very much. Overt and rigorous evaluation within most hospitals tends to be muted since their physicians are usually graduates of the same medical school. Covert evaluation of a physician's competence is made by peers, and by the public based on the hospital's prestige.[3]

Many Westerners, used to Japan's economic miracle, find it hard to accept just how mixed the quality of Japanese medical care really is. Not only are the best hospitals utterly congested, but the bulk of the small clinic/hospitals are physician-owned, profit-making institutions. (Any facility with more than 20 beds is a "hospital"; those with fewer than 20 beds are "clinics.") Public hospitals, though prestigious, are incredibly busy. Some chiefs of service, assisted by residents, see 100 people in a morning.[4] Forty percent of inpatients are over 65 years of age; half are hospitalized longer than six months. The average length of stay exceeds 40 days.[5]

In Japan the best-trained physicians do not, by any means, earn the most. The incomes of private practitioners fell from 8.2 times average wages in 1980 to 6.8 in 1987. Yet salaried physicians, including the best in academic positions, have incomes only 2.4 times average wages.[6] Moreover, the number of physicians has grown sharply, from 120 per 100,000 in 1976 to 157 per 100,000 in 1987.[7] Because nearly all that growth has occurred in urban areas, however, ample overall supply has not solved the problem of underdoctored rural areas.[8]

The serious issues go well beyond the quality of Japan's doctors and hospitals. The Japanese consume enormous amounts of prescription drugs; their per capita consumption is the highest in the world—about twice that of the United States[9]—and almost surely too high. A good part of the explanation is that Japanese doctors dispense drugs directly. They, in turn, buy drugs at a discount of about 25 percent on the fee

schedule and profit from the difference. This practice accounts for a
large part of medical incomes in Japan. (Since the early 1980s, health
insurers have pressed down on the pharmaceutical fee schedule, but
price declines have only increased the physicians' incentives to prescribe more.) In Japan, drug costs averaged just over 38 percent of
national medical expenditures in 1980. For clinics, more than 44 percent
of their income came from the prescription and dispensing of drugs.[10]
By contrast, in 1980, Americans spent 8.1 percent and in 1989, 7.4
percent of national health expenditures on prescription drugs.[11]

Even what appears to be sensible medical practice can get distorted
in the Japanese mix of economics and medicine. For example, the
Japanese fee schedule rewards ambulatory care and diagnostic procedures more than surgery. Indeed, there is something akin to a Japanese
aversion to surgery (with rates a quarter of ours, according to recent
estimates). On the other hand, there is a passion for diagnostic tests.
Japan has more advanced diagnostic tools (like CT scanners) than almost
any other country—"more a source of criticism," the *Economist* wrote
in 1990, "than of praise." With so much of the diagnostic equipment
owned by physicians, its use is an important source of medical income.
Patients no doubt get more tests than they need, and domestic manufacturers understandably concentrate on producing diagnostic equipment.[12] The result is that important innovations—like cardiac pace-
makers—are not produced locally and are much more expensive in
Japan than elsewhere. Japan has one of the highest kidney-dialysis rates
in the world, yet one of the lowest rates for organ transplants in general
and kidney transplants in particular.

Finally, Americans would be startled by conditions in the typical
Japanese hospital or clinic. Families do a lot of the nursing, and the
small institutions—more akin to diagnostic hotels and nursing homes
than modern medical centers—are nothing like the organizational wonders North Americans take for granted in their hospitals. The cramped
homes of Japan are reproduced in the hospital world and, for the Japanese who do not see the alternatives to their system, there is resigned
acceptance, not delight. Indeed, a six-nation opinion poll found the
Japanese to be the least satisfied with their medical care, with only 12
percent "very satisfied."[13]

Some external judgments are no less critical. "One lesson the Japanese experience teach[es] us," according to David Gross's probing review of Margaret Powell and Masahira Aneski's *Health Care in Japan*,[14]
"is that a disjointed delivery system, without adequate expenditure
controls, will lead to a proliferation of expensive technological equip-

ment, uncontrolled hospital growth, duplication of services, and increased volume in the presence of a payment system that encourages inefficient and excessive delivery of care."

This critique of Japanese medical care is sharply at odds with the celebrations of Western Japanophiles such as Norman MacRae, former editor of the influential *Economist,* who has claimed that "Japan's unplanned medical system is proving the most economic, with the best health delivery per few dollars spent." This, of course, mistakenly presumes that because the health results are good, the health care must be as well. "Lowest input," according to MacRae's reasoning, "brings best output." Wrong.

Healthy society, questionable medical care—what is one to think? How does Japan spend so little—about 7 percent of GNP, according to official figures[15]—and do so well by conventional health measures? The full answer requires a book-length discussion, but the short answer is simple. In the postwar period, the Japanese invested in a few crucial interventions—prenatal care, above all, is brilliantly managed as a public-health measure—and spent most of their energies getting wealthier. Despite what many Americans would regard as worrisome pollution, extraordinary stress (at work, at school and in transit), and severely cramped housing, the Japanese have absolutely fantastic health statistics without any experts believing the quality of their medical care is the main explanation. In fact, most epidemiologists account for Japan's comparative good health as largely the by-product of other things: the pride of real economic accomplishment, a deeply felt sense of social order, low levels of unemployment and high levels of education, all combined with a relatively more equal distribution of income, a good diet, and decent maternal and child health care.

Whatever its quality shortcomings, the accessibility and financing of Japanese medical care provide little basis for American smugness. Health insurance coverage is broad, reimbursement is tightly regulated, and the Japanese have financial access to the care available.

Health insurance coverage is based on employment and supplemented with government programs to fill in the gaps for uncovered groups. Japan gets to universal health insurance through the aggregation of separate programs, much like the German system on which it was modeled in the 1920s. Even though there is not one Japanese health scheme, the ground rules—for benefits, financing, fees, and eligibility—are dominated by the government. The sources of financing are multiple: roughly 60 percent from the employees' health insurance (public and private), 33 percent from the self-employed and pensioners' insurance plan, and 7 percent from the special geriatric pool. Nonetheless, Japan has been comparatively successful in restraining the share of their increasing wealth devoted to medical care. (Some analysts claim expenditures are understated, that if Japan measured its outlays as we do, the costs might constitute 9 percent of their gross national product— still low by our standards.)[16] Japan's most obvious shortcoming is its quality of medical care, not the level or sources of medical financing.

Nor is the problem with Japanese medical care one of sheer access. There are plenty of medical facilities and ample numbers of clinicians, and universal health insurance has removed the economic barriers to care. With the use of hospitals and clinics unrestricted by finances, Japan has the highest rate of outpatient consultation in the world. With emergency care readily accessible, Japanese commentators can also say that their citizens have easy access to care when accidents strike. Indeed, according to a national survey, of those who had experienced an illness but had not seen physicians, only 0.4 percent gave economic reasons for not doing so, and most said the problem was not serious.[17] Nor is relatively equal access a pipe dream. It is, for example, illegal for providers to demand extra payment other than for hospital room charges and a very restricted range of specialized services. In fact, hospitals cannot legally offer better food for patients in private rooms.

No one sensibly attributes the Japanese achievement in longevity and infant mortality to Japan's quite uneven medical care. But all the experts, while acknowledging that socioeconomic and dietary factors play the major role, point to Japan's maternal and child services as very important. The Japanese made prenatal care one of their top medical priorities, and the payoff has been substantial. How do they do it? First, Japan provides free and unlimited medical exams to all pregnant women, infants, and young children. Second, Japan has universal health insurance for maternity and infant care services. Third, Japan's medical clinics provide guidance classes for pregnant women, who are generally well educated and receptive. Fourth, midwives and nurses make regular home visits to pregnant women and women with infants. Fifth, family-planning counseling is widely available.

By contrast, the United States is appallingly bad at assuring basic care to all pregnant women. As the Children's Defense Fund reports, "After many years of substantial progress, our nation's improvement in the rates of early prenatal care, low-birth-weight births, and infant mortality has slowed down dramatically or stopped. Immunization rates actually have declined. The United States has slipped to nineteenth in the world in preventing infant deaths, behind such nations as Spain,

Ireland, Hong Kong and Singapore." The United States now ranks twentieth in the world in infant mortality, twenty-ninth in low-birth-weight babies, and fifteenth in polio immunization.

Despite Japan's clear success in reducing maternal and infant mortality, the broader lessons of its health and medical performance are decidedly ambiguous. While Japan's medical spending is comparatively low, the rate of increase in per capita outlays from 1972 to 1992 was, as in the United States, very rapid. The costs of Japan's medical care are held down—to the extent that they are—by a powerful set of negotiating rules and limits on fees. On the delivery side, the Japanese example is one largely of laissez-faire. This combination of unrestrained delivery arrangements and highly discordant bargaining over fees has worked tolerably well so far. But the Japanese have not found a way—through effective but acceptable regional planning—to constrain the supply of services and physicians and thus to reduce the extraordinary reliance on fee negotiations to control medical costs.

Finally, Japan, like the United States, has experienced sharp increases in its elderly population. The Japanese focus on the hospital provides no model of independent living for the frail or chronically ill older person capable, with assistance, of living at home.

Even more important, the Japanese experience suggests that improving the quality of medical care may not be all that important to health. Japan's really startling lesson is that its sharply improved health status has not—with the major exception of care for mothers and infants—depended on medical improvements. But if diet, economic success, high levels of education, and a sense of social cohesion *appear* crucial to Japan's healthiness, how helpful is their example? Our grandmothers all knew these lessons, but it is much harder to change such basic features of American society than to fill every hospital in the land with MRI equipment and the like. Japan's medical care may be a mixed bag, but the country's healthiness is remarkable and especially sobering for us Americans—preoccupied with health and medical care to what is probably an unhealthy degree.

Part IV

Policy Choices: Dilemmas and Decisions

Chapter 14
Coalition or Collision?
Medicare and Health Reform

As Chapter 9 noted, the reform of American medicine rose to the top of the public agenda by 1992 with remarkable speed and support. Yet there is no assurance that the rare agreement on the nation's medical ills will generate the legislative backing required for a substantively adequate, workable program of reform.

The agenda President Clinton proposed could not possibly have been specified in detail from his campaign. As a campaigner, he understandably avoided concentrating on the details of health policy or its implementation. As President, however, he has different opportunities and risks. In health, he must specify workable means to his reform aims that can command a majority in the Congress.

That task is one of the most difficult a presidential reformer faces. We have seen that reformers in the Progressive era and the New Deal, under President Truman, and during the early 1970s thought universal health insurance was imminent and were bitterly disappointed. Now, as then, entrenched interests try to block change by skillfully manipulating our deepest fears and beliefs to maintain their privileges. In 1993, to be sure, those interests seemed to be on the defensive; the time for reform does appear to have arrived. But before the new administration and the

Reprinted by permission from *American Prospect* 12 (Winter 1993), pp. 53–59.
Copyright © 1993, New Prospect, Inc.

Congress can resolve the challenges of reform, they will have to resolve
some nasty and hardly trivial budget problems stemming from Medicare
and other current federal health programs. The stage is set for what
could become a nightmare of conflicting agendas.

CAP SNAP

We had a premonition of conflicts to come in July 1992, when
budget director Richard Darman predicted that Medicare outlays would
have to be drastically reduced to cut the budget deficit. Hence Darman
proposed a "cap" on Medicare and Medicaid to reduce federal health
spending between 1993 and 1997 by some $260 billion. In response,
candidate Clinton charged that such a policy would eviscerate federal
health programs. Kenneth E. Thorpe, an economist advising the Clinton
campaign, warned that enforcing such caps without more far-reaching
medical care reforms would destroy Medicaid, increase cost-shifting
from Medicare to employment-based insurance, and thus lead to the
loss of millions of jobs. The Bush campaign claimed this was nothing
but the familiar scare tactics of Democrats. Nonetheless, Bush tried to
distance himself from the flareup by calling Darman's proposal merely
one option.

As President, Clinton cannot easily escape the problem that Darman
identified. It will be no easy matter for his administration to deal with
Medicare and its constituencies while taking steps toward universal
health insurance and a transformation of how we pay for and deliver
medical care. If the Clinton plan fails to incorporate the elderly, and
quickly, Medicare is at political and fiscal risk in the interim. The danger
here is a potentially serious clash between the constituencies of Medicare and of universal health insurance and the reawakening of the ugly
generational politics that marked the debacle over Medicare catastrophic coverage—the program that Congress enacted in 1988 only to
repeal the following year after an eruption of discontent from the affluent
elderly.

Were it possible to enact universal health insurance immediately and
to fold Medicare into such a program, a generational conflict would not
necessarily arise. But universal health insurance simply may not proceed that fast. Clinton himself has signaled as much. His aim is to reach
universal coverage by several transitional steps, meanwhile setting in
place the elements of overall cost control. He has proposed requiring
employers to pay for health insurance, with public financing for the
unemployed, and suggested folding Medicaid beneficiaries as well as

some of the employed into health insurance purchasing groups. President Clinton's hope, quite clearly, is to produce by the end of his first term a coherent amalgam of the fragmented arrangements we euphemistically call the American health care system. But what about Medicare in the here and now?

Although Medicare's costs are now growing as rapidly as those of private insurance, they pose major budgetary problems. Compared with other federal programs, Medicare's 30 percent growth in cost in four years makes it one of the most rapidly expanding items in the budget. Hence Budget Director Darman's talk of capping Medicare's expenditure increases. But any attempt to do so, without controls on the rest of the health economy, would exacerbate one of the worst trends in health finance during the 1980s: the shifting of Medicare expenses from public accounts to private insurance and patient bills.

If Clinton intends to make good on his promise to cut half the budget deficit by 1996, he will have to show how Medicare outlays will be constrained. After all, the economic plan he released during the campaign presumed "savings" of scores of billions of Medicare outlays over the Bush administration's fearful forecasts that uncapped Medicare expenditures would grow at 15.8 percent annually. Those savings must come from either reductions in what Medicare pays or increased Medicare taxes, or both.

To get savings amounting to $145 billion over this period, the Bush administration proposed what amount to draconian burdens on our elderly, our hospitals, and some of our physicians. A quick review makes plain why Darman's proposed cap excited such outrage. To save nearly $64 billion in Medicare's physician insurance program, Bush proposed increases in the premiums and cost-sharing for which the elderly are responsible. Such changes, the Congressional Budget Office estimated, would, along with increased payments for supplementary private policies, raise the elderly's spending on medical care from 7 percent of their incomes to nearly 12 percent by 1997. Other proposed spending cuts in physician coverage ($14 billion over five years) presumed reductions in payments to doctors.

Additional savings, estimated at $68.8 billion, would come from Medicare's hospital program. Today Medicare pays something like 90 percent of reported hospital costs. Bush proposed to pay hospitals about 72 percent of their costs by 1992. On the basis of past experience, hospitals would expect to shift much of those reductions to other payers. Thus, spending cuts in Medicare alone would likely mean higher medical bills for the elderly (cost-shifting backward), increased burdens on employers (cost-shifting sideways), and decreased revenues or higher fees for physicians (cost-shifting forward). Such a policy would enrage those groups and complicate enormously any more fundamental reform of the way American medical care is organized and financed.

The short-run problem facing Clinton is obvious. Medicare appears a voracious consumer of public dollars. On its present course, an unreformed Medicare seems certain to defeat hopes for deficit reduction. How can the Clinton administration get Medicare's outlays under control without the full fright (and fight) sketched above?

At its inception in 1965, Medicare was seen as a way to bring the elderly into the mainstream of American medicine. Its hospital coverage and medical insurance mirrored the dominant forms of Blue Cross/Blue Shield and commercial health insurance in the postwar period. For more than fifteen years, the program's cost grew rapidly, rising from 9.2 percent of national health expenditures in 1967 to 16.7 percent in 1984. During this period the program paid hospitals "reasonable costs" and physicians "reasonable and customary fees." But the unreasonable result was that Medicare helped to promote seemingly uncontrollable health care inflation.

Since the mid-1980s, however, the Medicare program has had far less rapid growth than medical care generally. Few people are aware of it, but the facts are undeniable: the rate of increase in Medicare outlays fell sharply from an average of 16 percent between 1980 and 1985 to an average of 9 percent between 1986 and 1990. The increase in outlays for 1991 was only 6.3 percent (Table 14.1).

As Marilyn Moon, a health care analyst at the Urban Institute, shows in her 1993 book, *Medicare Now and the Future,* Medicare controlled its costs more tightly than did private health insurers during this same period. Despite the fiscal strain of the recent recession and the undeniable cost-shifting that Medicare has prompted, its health budget pressures are less than those facing American businesses and workers. The fearsome picture of Medicare's future stems from the rapid inflation officially projected for the rest of the 1990s. For example, the Congressional Budget Office estimates that Medicare outlays will increase at approximately 11 percent every year from 1993 through 1997.

WHAT COULD A RESPONSIBLE
ADMINISTRATION DO?

The Bush administration's answer to rising Medicare costs was to cut Medicare benefits and reimbursement rates and to increase costs

Table 14.1
Medicare outlays, fiscal years 1980–1991

Year	Total outlay (in billions)	Percent increase
1980	35,025	20.1
1981	42,488	21.3
1982	50,424	18.7
1983	56,935	12.9
1984	62,480	9.7
1985	71,384	14.3
1986	75,903	6.3
1987	81,640	7.6
1988	87,677	7.4
1989	96,555	10.1
1990	109,709	13.6
1991	116,657	6.3

Source: 1992 Green Book, House Ways and Means Committee, p. 189.

to the elderly. The alternative is to restructure Medicare, and American health care more generally, to put both on a more affordable trajectory. But the hardest questions remain: which strategy of reform to choose, and what steps are required for implementation?

One strategy would be to reform Medicare as a first step in the process of making the transition to national cost controls and universal coverage. That goal presumes that Medicare expenditures simply cannot be permitted to grow at rates of 11 to 15 percent per year. So, by "Medicare reform" I mean two things. The first is to restrict Medicare's budget growth to a rate comparable to general inflation, not twice that; the second is to embrace a program of long-term care and catastrophic coverage to relieve the legitimate anxieties of the elderly.

Restraining the rate of Medicare's current budget growth would head off some of the direct conflict among Medicare and universal health insurance constituents, provided that cost controls were imposed throughout the medical economy and precluded another orgy of cost-shifting. The generality of the cost controls—not whether national expenditure limits are enforced through price and volume controls or produced through managed competition—is the crucial element in this approach.

Such reforms require incorporating Medicare's constituencies into the demand for overall cost control. It is here that the clash of generational politics is most dangerous. To avoid that means a serious commitment to relieving the continuing health worries of the elderly.

To reform Medicare as part of the transition to national cost controls and universal coverage offers a difficult politics. We need to acknowledge honestly the elderly's fears of economic insecurity from the costs of catastrophic illness and long-term care. To address those problems requires adding to Medicare by the end of 1996 a social insurance program covering long-term care and catastrophic medical expenses. This, of course, raises the risk of the legislative disaster acted out over Medicare catastrophic coverage in 1988–1989. On the other hand, the linking of increased benefits to earmarked social insurance taxes has considerably more popular support than the oft-cited American aversion to taxes would suggest. A 1988 survey reported that 63 percent of Americans favor increasing access to medical care rather than lowering the nation's health spending.

The long-term care and catastrophic proposals raise somewhat different issues. Long-term care is not an ordinary medical matter, and there are legitimate disputes over whether it should be part of health insurance at all. What is not in dispute is that Americans fear impoverishment from frailty in old age; the dread of Alzheimer's disease has universalized this anxiety. No system of private insurance—without cross-subsidization and extensive regulation—can spread the financial risks of long-term frailty widely enough to be affordable to those with modest incomes. Social insurance, with small payments spread out over a lifetime of work, is precisely the risk-spreading device called for in such circumstances. As with catastrophic protection against the costs of acute care, the burden of financing should be distributed over both time and income classes. An increase in Medicare taxes so justified would be far more compelling than nonearmarked tax increases, the polls (and common sense) tell us.

The political disaster that resulted when catastrophic insurance was repealed because the elderly resented paying for it entirely themselves was not the result of taking on the wrong problem. Rather, an analysis reveals calculated misinformation, poor legislative design of an otherwise sound program's financing, and ill-managed politics (see Table 14.2). The "rationale behind the ill-fated Medicare catastrophic coverage legislation was compelling and remains compelling in the aftermath of

Table 14.2
*Medicare spending under current policy and under proposed Bush
administration cap (in billions)*

Year	Baseline	Entitlement cap
1993	$146.1	$139.2
1994	163.6	148.8
1995	182.8	156.2
1996	204.9	163.6
1997	228.1	170.8

Source: President's midsession review, July 24, 1992.

its repeal," Edward Lawlor of the University of Chicago has rightly
argued.

The disaster was largely the result of departing from social insurance
principles of finance, concentrating tax increases solely on the current
elderly, and failing to explain why that choice made sense, particularly
to the more comfortable elderly with their own supplementary policies.
The experience offers a lesson for reform. Both for catastrophic protection against the costs of acute illness and for the social and economic
problems of long-term care, social insurance financing makes most
sense. Administering either will be difficult, and the political fears each
will excite are considerable. But there is reward here as well as risk.

The reward would be a dampening of the fears of elderly constituents
and their pressure groups about their interests being sacrificed in budget
deficit struggles and the transition to universal health insurance. However, meeting these concerns of the elderly also may reignite the political
hostility toward the elderly evident in the battle over Medicare catastrophic. Two decades of fiscal strain have worsened intergenerational
strains in American public life.

Because our welfare state has concentrated on programs for the
elderly—as with social security pensions and Medicare—welfare state
critics have seized on the image of "greedy geezers" as the explanation
for our woes. The scapegoating, led by the Americans for Generational
Equity and supported by Wall Street gurus like Peter Peterson, is an
unanticipated consequence of how we have structured our public house-
hold. Canada, for instance, has a nearly identical proportion of elderly
citizens and similar rates of medical care use by its elderly; it also
experienced comparable economic strain during the 1970s and 1980s.

But its universal medical program addresses the sick, not the elderly, so Canada has nothing comparable to our hand-wringing about the "graying of the federal budget."

The implication is that we should address the real problems facing the elderly while taking deliberate steps to incorporate their health insurance into a wider, less age-graded system. Convincing the Congress that this is both possible and desirable will not be easy. Many will remember the catastrophic episode bitterly, buttressed by the image of Congressman Dan Rostenkowski being hounded on a Chicago street by what amounted to a mob of older Americans. A presidential commitment to addressing Medicare reform while moving toward universal health insurance would help enormously. Making sure that the controls on cost bring genuine savings, not cost shifting from Medicare, is crucial. The task of designing that transition is an unheralded but central element in the new administration's agenda.

Such reform, of course, is easier to propose than to produce. Could we reform Medicare as suggested above and simultaneously place a budget limit on overall health expenditures? Could we at the same time add a program for pregnant women and children, thus addressing one of our most pressing needs in access? And could we also address the concerns about financial disaster for the uninsured and underinsured by a temporary program of refundable tax credits for medical expenses beyond, for example, 15 percent of annual income? No one would want such a program permanently, but as a stopgap isn't it administratively workable and relatively free of bureaucratic complexity?

These are questions, not firm answers. With budget limits, improved access in stages, and time to augment America's supply of capitated health care systems, these proposals are worth raising while admitting uncertainty about their feasibility. Most important, such transitions attend to political fissures that exist quite beyond the traditional opposition to the combination of universal health insurance and cost controls among private insurers and their allies.

This approach to incremental reform brings enormous risks of misinformation. None of the elderly constituencies will be fooled by vague promises of attending to Medicare after introducing a new program for those under age 65 built on principles different from Medicare's. It is worth sketching out an alternative scenario.

The most appealing, yet difficult approach would be to introduce simultaneously a national budget for medical care and an insurance program for all those under 65. As Clinton has suggested, a national health care commission would set a budget limit for expenditures, allocate subnational limits to the states, and hold Medicare to a specified share of that budget. These are daunting tasks of implementation, but the general idea would be to incorporate Medicare budget constraints into an overall cap on health expenditures and to fold Medicare into the decentralized administration of cost control planned for the nation as a whole.

If the Congress enacted universal coverage by aggregating separate programs for the employed, the unemployed, veterans, the poor, and Medicare, the result would be administratively complex. Play-or-pay plans would require not only budget limits, but state rate setting to control the pressures on expenditures. Evidence from the 1970s and 1980s, developed by Thorpe, shows that states which implemented rate setting had rates of medical inflation comparable to Canada's. But such programs would have to cover all health insurance plans within a state, and Medicare would have to be incorporated in such efforts. The appeal to the elderly constituencies would arise from the benefit additions suggested above, with the funds drawn from earmarked Medicare taxes spread over the entire working population and increased Medicare premiums. Were the Congress to mandate universal coverage for those under 65 on terms commonly described as "managed competition," other options for Medicare remain. One approach, as Paul Starr suggested in his book *The Logic of Health-Care Reform,* would be to offer the new program as an option to people older than 65. This alternative could be made attractive to many now in Medicare with the inclusion of catastrophic coverage, and the new program might very well become mandatory for new cohorts reaching age 65. On that model, Medicare itself would fade away over time.

In each of these options, the central political feature is that Medicare beneficiaries are promised improvements in their circumstances as part of a broader health care reform. Under some, the program continues but is subject to administrative cost controls on the entire medical care industry. Many analysts doubt whether such administered prices can work well in an industry as complex and changing as medical care. But we have ample experience from Canada and Australia that countervailing public power can restrain medical inflation more readily than our current system. Whether the prospects of price and volume controls are better than the promise of managed competition is a question no one can answer with confidence. Nearly two decades of managed care programs should leave no one smug about those prospects. Managed competition has never been tried comprehensively and, necessarily, cannot be said to have been proven in practice. Whether through monopsony bargaining over budgets, rates, and allocations or through a decentralized system of health maintenance organizations, the double task for health care reform is to dampen medical inflation while widening access. I suggest that options exist to do so without reenacting the generational warfare that marked the ill-fated catastrophic reforms of the late 1980s.

One such option, seemingly the most straightforward, would subsume medical care for the elderly under the new universal plan; Medicare as a separate program would cease to exist. This option, however, has three necessary preconditions. First, the basic benefits of the universal program would have to be at least as comprehensive as Medicare's current physician and hospital coverage; second, its administration would have to be simpler and more responsive; and third, the new universal plan would have to be implemented speedily enough so that Medicare would not continue to bleed red ink during a long interim.

There are valuable lessons we can draw from the frustrations of the past two decades. One is that the opportunities for reform are few and precious, not to be squandered. The excellent but undoable should not be allowed to defeat what is both good and doable. Another is that piecemeal change, without a clear timetable, design, and commitment to where one wants to get, is both frustrating and politically wasteful. There is no easy escape from addressing problems simultaneously, even if the steps of reform must be sequenced. Cost control without increased access to health insurance was a disaster in the late 1970s. Expanding access without reforming the financial structure of American medicine is no better, as the catastrophic debacle illustrates. But reforming Medicare while moving toward universal financial coverage and workable restraints on health expenditures should be within our grasp.

Chapter 15
Implementation:
Making Reform Work

No one seriously doubts that American health care needs reform. Although the language of crisis is undoubtedly overused in American politics, there is now a widely shared conviction that costs in our health care system are too high compared to the benefits received, that too many citizens have no health insurance or inadequate insurance, and that the complexity of our financing and reimbursement arrangements bedevils patients, payers, and providers to an insufferable degree. These complaints—which together have produced what sociologist Paul Starr has rightly called a "negative consensus"[1]—have brought reform to the very top of the American political agenda. President Clinton came to office partly on the basis of his promise to fix this mess. And the fate of the Clinton presidency will rest to a considerable degree on its effectiveness in addressing the problems on which a negative consensus exists.

Unfortunately, the debate about potential remedies for these problems has satisfied almost no one. Labels and symbols of proposals, not real standards for their assessment, have dominated the discussion. The unprecedented and extensive efforts of the President's Task Force on Health Care Reform—partly because of an understandable preference

Reprinted by permission from *Domestic Affairs* (Winter, 1993/94), pp. 143–57.

for private deliberations—have not clarified the central principles by which the administration's plan, or its competitors, should be judged.

Broad approaches are typically identified, in Washingtonese shorthand, as "managed competition," "single-payer," or "tax-credit" reform plans. These tags are for some purposes reasonable, highlighting important similarities and distinctions among proposals. But if such categories illuminate, they also obscure. Classification, by its very nature, stresses differences across groups and similarities within them—and therefore tends to ignore or understate similarities across groups and differences within them. At the same time, perfervid discussions of rumors and leaks regularly focus attention on stupifyingly complex details without contributing to, or proceeding from, a coherent sense of how the competing values of cost control, accessibility, flexibility, and quality assurance ought to be pursued and balanced. And withal, one fundamental set of issues consistently gets short shrift: how, and how well, would alternative policy options actually be implemented if they were to be adopted?

THE CENTRALITY OF IMPLEMENTATION

Others have discussed the variety of standards by which competing proposals for reform will be judged. The focus of this chapter will be implementation—a topic that is crucial to wise policy choice as well as to improved administration. After all, it would not be sensible to assume that one reform plan is superior to another merely because it falls into one category or another; the particulars of a plan—the chances that it would prove workable—ought to weigh heavily in our judgment of it. We need to move beyond our preconceptions of plans to realistic forecasts of their implementation.

Suppose, for example, that we compare two hypothetical proposals— one a single-payer scheme, the other a procompetitive design. And suppose that both appear promising in theory, but on closer analysis, we surmise that the first, as a consequence of its detailed features, would be likely to result in a poorly structured, badly managed single-payer program—a Medicaid fantasy writ large—and that the second, again based on specifics of its design, seems likely to yield a carefully and skillfully regulated program of managed competition in which patient-consumers choose from among a few high-quality, nationwide plans (much as they do now with long-distance telephone companies.) No responsible advocate of Canadian-style, single-payer health care reform, however committed to this ideal, would favor the first proposal, given its practical ineffectiveness. Conversely, if we were to compare a well-worked-out single-payer plan with a poorly conceived managed competition scheme, no thoughtful proponent of market-based reform, however intense his or her commitment to that theory, would favor the latter.

To be successful, any reform effort—whatever the "approach" it seems to correspond to—will require skilled government regulation and oversight. Yet this fact of reform is often overlooked by advocates of all sorts of plans. On the one hand, managed competition (and play-or-pay) advocates frequently minimize the extent of government supervision required to make their plans work well. On the other hand, proponents of single-payer reform too often fail to address genuine concerns about government's capability to manage such a system.

The tendency to overlook implementation issues is not surprising, given how difficult, and unglamorous, it is to figure out the nuts and bolts of real programs—and how much more enticing it is for politicians and policy analysts to bandy about big ideas. The implementation of policy is less visible and less dramatic than the framing of policy—and often, frankly, more arcane. The neglect of implementation issues is more than a simple intellectual mistake; it may also be a rational response to the fact that our political system confers more rewards for the shrewd deployment of symbols and generalized arguments than it does for detailed, realistic analysis and forecasting.

When initially considering the implementation of any new program, one is immediately aware of all the complexity (and uncertainty) involved. This is especially true of health care reform. Carrying out major changes in an industry that will consume $930 billion in 1993—nearly one-seventh of the American economy—is an undeniably formidable task.

But the implementation issues involved in sustaining the status quo are no less formidable: the complex processes by which 14 percent of GNP is raised now; the extraordinary range of administrative activities through which doctors, hospitals, drug firms, nursing homes, health maintenance organizations, and utilization review companies are paid; and the diverse means by which capital for expansion, renovation, and innovation is raised and allocated. The question, then, is not simply what tasks are daunting, but which ones are both desirable *and* doable.

Let us consider, then, two of the most important policy choices facing reformers—how best to control and distribute costs and how best to distribute administrative authority and complexity—and explore the implementation issues involved in each. Needless to say, these topics do not cover the full range of implementation issues raised by national health care reform. However, they do raise undeniably important questions for such reform, and they illustrate the significance of paying close attention to implementation.

COST CONTROL: ASPIRATION AND IMPLEMENTATION

Most reformers (and reform plans) aspire to constrain the spiraling costs of American health care, but they disagree substantially on how to achieve that common end. The choice, according to many, is between market-based and government-based strategies, between "competition" and "regulation." As I have written elsewhere,[2] this is a false and misleading dichotomy.

It is unrealistic to suppose either that we would move to wholly unfettered competition in the provision of health care in this country or that any conceivable form of government health program would eradicate competition—for patients, prestige, and honor—among doctors, hospitals, and health care organizations. This much President Clinton acknowledged in his frequent references to competition within the context of a global budget. But what implementation issues do we need to think through in considering the expanded use of competitive health plans and the imposition of global budgets?

For proponents of competition, the task appears easy: more incentives, less government. Al From, who heads the Democratic Leadership Council, recently explained what a "new Democrat" would prefer in the way of a health care reform plan. First, reform "should not resort to government price controls or sweeping employer mandates." And second, it should involve phasing in "both universal coverage and a tough form of managed competition to discipline the demand for care in the face of expanding coverage, by requiring nearly everyone to take more financial responsibility for his or her own medical care."[3]

There is much one might say about the substantive merits of a "tough form of managed competition," and even more about what could be meant by the suggestion that patients take "more financial responsibility." Putting all of that to one side, what basis is there for forecasting successful implementation of either of these elements?

There is, of course, no agreed-upon design for "managed competition," tough or tame. The core notions include the following. Citizens would choose among competing health insurance plans, all of which would be required to offer at least a common, basic benefit package.

Plans would compete in part by offering coverage beyond the basic package, but any additional costs—whether for extra benefits or, in some variants of managed competition, for the incremental cost of higher-priced basic packages—would have to be paid with after-tax income. These arrangements are intended to generate restraint in the purchase of coverage and, because of the potential that enrollees would exit from unsatisfactory plans, inducements for managers to bargain hard with providers and to satisfy their "customers." How likely is it that proposals of this sort would have their desired effects?

The only reasonable answer is a skeptical one. Policymakers would have to discount heavily the benefits presumed to follow from adopting such an innovative strategy for controlling health care costs. The desirability of this strategy depends on the interests to which insurance plans are actually responsive, the ability of the general public to control the behavior of competing plans, and the implications of that behavior for more equal access and more restrained expenditures. As others have noted,[4] the expected behavior of insurance firms (whether paying for care or also organizing care in provider networks) raises problems on all counts.

Requirements for open enrollment and public subsidies that vary with risk—prerequisites for a managed competition approach to reform—aim to eliminate current restrictions on the availability of insurance for high-risk individuals. But such provisions will not eliminate the rewards to insurance plans for avoiding expensive customers unless they are accompanied by a comprehensive specification of high risks. That in turn is a difficult and highly controversial task, one never accomplished on a national scale. Indeed, where risk-adjusted capitation rates have been attempted—in the Netherlands, for example—the task has proved administratively costly and exceedingly complex.[5] This experience hardly provides grounds for assuming that competing plans will vie for clients on socially acceptable bases.

There are many ways that plans can maintain selective memberships. One is to exclude people by manipulating the availability of services. Organizations providing care can make themselves inconvenient and unattractive to the elderly by offering poor services for those with chronic illnesses, or they can find locations that attract statistically low-risk populations—for example, in high-income suburbs rather than urban ghettos. To achieve similar effects, plans may well restrict coverage to particular physicians—a practice that would not leave high-risk persons without insurance, but that would increase the cost of providing their care and strain the resources of the plans that serve them. This sorting of patients by risk would obviously conflict with equitable sharing of the costs of illness.

In any effort to adjust for relative risks, the more detailed the actuarial categories used and the more precise the relationships between categories and subsidies, the less likely and extensive the resultant inequities. But detail and precision are costly in multiple ways. They increase administrative complexity and expense—and at the same time they require greater oversight of provider and insurer practices. What might seem relatively straightforward could in practice be anything but.

These are the most obvious of the gaps between promise and likely performance in an untried system of managed competition.[6] The very fact that no nation in the world has tried such an approach is cause for discounting the promised benefits. Our judgments as to whether the likely results would be worse or better than those of alternative strategies ought to depend on comparative forecasts, not ideological promises.

Those promoting the cost-control potential of so-called single-payer models are in a somewhat different position regarding implementation. They can argue, on the basis of operational experience in many OECD countries, that their preferred strategy is doable. The evidence is unmistakable that nations with concentrated forms of health care financing—however complex in institutional detail—have in fact demonstrated greater cost restraint than the United States. That much can be inferred from the clustering of health expenditures around 8 to 9 percent of GNP in nations as different from each other as Germany, France, Canada, and Australia.[7]

It is one thing to note evidence of the operational possibility of such cost control and another to forecast what its implementation would be like in the United States. On this point, the indications are mixed. Cost control in practice requires a combination of political will, administrative capability, and effective means. Single-payer systems, using a variety of payment and budget devices, have proved effective when joined to administratively capable and motivated governmental (or quasi-governmental) units.

In the United States, the Medicare program proved able in the late 1980s to reduce its rate of expenditure increases below that of the health insurance industry as a whole.[8] In addition, the Medicaid program has shown the will and the capacity to sharply restrict physician fees and hospital payments, holding them below what providers regard as tolerable. But the problem with drawing inferences from such partial "successes" is obvious. These exercises in cost control affect only some segments of the American public, allowing the shifting of costs to others. We cannot from this experience unambiguously predict the extent to which overall U.S. costs would be controlled in a single-payer system. However, this track record does provide grounds for believing it likely that either the federal government or the states, facing global limits and pressures from other claimants on public funds, could enforce such limits. It is beyond the ambit of this discussion to inquire whether such enforcement might produce side effects more worrisome than health care inflation. Regarding cost control, however, we do have a basis for predicting a larger gap between promise and likely performance in managed competition programs than in Medicare-like single-payer schemes.

COMPLEXITY: DISTRIBUTION AND REDUCTION

Reformers of every persuasion are united in wanting less complexity (and cost) in the administration of health insurance. American health care, it is agreed, should be much simpler than the system we now have. Its rules should be comprehensible. Patients and providers alike ought to know how to use the system, where to complain, and whom to blame if something goes wrong.

Nevertheless, the yearning for greater simplicity has not produced sophisticated debate about how to achieve it. Indeed, this topic is woefully underdiscussed in terms of either policy or implementation. Simplicity in operation, of course, requires simplicity of design. If all Americans are covered under basically the same terms, a simple national health insurance card should work. National standards that all plans must meet should assure portability of benefits. Simpler coverage allows simpler billing. But simplicity is not just a matter of insurance design; it is also a matter of administrative design.

The challenge is to sort out and distribute the tasks of administration so as to reduce complexity where that is possible—and where complexity is unavoidable, to place it on appropriate parties. For this sort of analysis, distinguishing proposals on the basis of whether they include single or multiple insurance plans is only a beginning point—and a potentially misleading one at that. The central issue is who bears what burdens in the daily operation of health insurance.

Consider, for illustrative purposes, a health insurance program that is undeniably simple for patients to use. There is one plan in a state, the benefits of which cover what everyone considers ordinary hospital and physician services. Patients tender the equivalent of a credit card to their caregivers and, except for hospital bills that cover extras such as a private room, that is the end of the administrative transaction from the patients' perspective. Hospitals face an annual budget negotiated in advance and receive monthly payments. Physicians' offices file computer reports on the care they provide, which indicate each patient's identification number, the code of the service rendered, and the date of service; payment arrives within three weeks. The insurance organization negotiates hospital and physician budgets—a controversial matter—and routinely pays each hospital the monthly allocation of its annual budget and each doctor his or her fees according to an agreed-upon schedule that does not permit extra or so-called balance billing. All of this is possible, we know, because I have just described with 95 percent accuracy what happens in the universal health insurance programs of both Canada and Australia.

Simplicity from the standpoints of patients and payments does not mean such systems are simple to operate. The single plan acts as a cooperative for patients, relieving them of paperwork, payments when they are sick, and hassles over who is to pay for what. This shifts such matters to the insurance program, rather than eliminating them. To be sure, it is easier (even if conflictual) to negotiate an operating budget for a hospital than to figure out the payments for individual services or diagnoses, as with American diagnosis-related group (DRG) hospital payments. Negotiations require talent, knowledge, and bargaining skills that are never in ample supply. Having one plan economizes, of course, on the talent search, but it is worth bearing in mind how much administrative capacity is required to run a single plan well. For that reason we should be spending much more time investigating alternatives to ordinary government departments in health insurance reform; we might well want to invent medical equivalents of the Federal Reserve, an organization with a public function that draws its talented officials from a very wide pool and has more freedom to reward them than does the typical federal, state, or local department.

Consider, by contrast, what would be involved in setting up institutions of managed competition. For some patients, having a limited number of plans from which to choose would be simpler than the options they now face. But for most, the choices would be difficult; the evidence of experience is that Americans overwhelmingly yearn for prepayment of medical bills, not choices among plans. The federal government employee plan is a good illustration of current complexity; it offers so many choices that consulting firms have sprung up to assist employees. Multiple plans, especially self-administration by large, nationwide employers, would complicate monitoring. Two-worker families could well face different terms of coverage—especially different doctors and hospitals in competing health alliances. This is not to suggest that such a scheme is without merit. Rather, it is to emphasize that multiple plans present patients with more complexity than much simpler alternative arrangements.

From the perspective of providers, a managed competition scheme would reduce complexity in some respects and increase it in others. The establishment of one clearinghouse through which to buy coverage—whether it is called a health insurance purchasing cooperative or something else—is a relocation of the role played by health departments in systems like Canada's. Each of these clearinghouses would have to negotiate with doctors and hospitals, but not directly. Competing health insurance plans would negotiate contracts with providers, not budgets for hospitals or fees for physicians. It is evident that such arrangements, while less complex than some current practices, are far less straightforward than single-plan health insurance.

From the perspective of payers, the forecast is more difficult. We have thus far not mentioned the greatest implementation barrier to managed competition: the absence in much of rural America of alternative sources of care that could be arranged in competing plans. Depending on the number of buying cooperatives, payers could face either a single institution (what you would expect in South Dakota, for example) or many intermediaries. Given that we now have 1,500 health insurance carriers in the United States, payers on average could expect considerably fewer. We know from German experience that multiple payers are manageable and, indeed, can coordinate their terms of payment.

The other sources of complexity in national health care reform are many. If a standard benefit package were to exclude what most would regard as ordinary medical care, boundary disputes would necessarily arise and make operations more complicated. If states are to be given a major role in administering universal health insurance, interstate negotiations would be required. The extent and character of utilization review, policies for reimbursement, the regulation of capital, initiatives to affect the supply and distribution of providers—these and literally scores of other aspects of reform could raise thorny issues of implementation.

The purpose of this discussion has been to illustrate how and where gaps between policy and performance are likely to arise, not to emphasize major cleavages in the public debate over health care reform. What seems clear is that in order to make wise choices, policymakers need to anticipate likely operational disappointments; they need to demand, and rely on, realistic implementation forecasts. Otherwise, we could end up with policies that are appealing in theory but appalling in practice.

Notes

CHAPTER 1: AMERICAN HEALTH CARE REFORM

1. This is a commonplace in the polling literature. See, e.g., Robert Blendon and Karen Donelan, "The Public and the Emerging Debate over National Health Insurance," *New England Journal of Medicine,* Vol. 323, No. 3 (1990), pp. 208–12.
2. See Theodore R. Marmor and Andrew Dunham, "The Politics of Health Policy Reform: Origins, Alternatives, and a Possible Prescription," in *Health Care: How to Improve it and Pay for It* (Washington, D.C.: Center for National Policy, 1985).
3. The Glossary explains the technical meaning of these jargon terms as used in the health reform debate.
4. For the developments in the 1970s, see Judy Feder, John Holohan, and Theodore R. Marmor, eds., *National Health Insurance: Conflicting Goals and Policy Choices* (Washington, D.C.: Urban Institute Press, 1980), Introduction.
5. See Mark Goldberg and Theodore R. Marmor, ". . . And What the Experts Expect: Among Health Care Factions, a Common Ground Is Emerging," *Washington Post,* Outlook Section, February 14, 1993.
6. This section draws extensively on Goldberg and Marmor, ". . . And What the Experts Expect."
7. Report by Robert Pear in the *New York Times,* April 10, 1993.
8. As outlined in Paul Starr's *Logic of Health Care Reform* (Nashville, Tenn.: Whittle Publications, 1993). Starr was, it should be noted, one of the key architects of *the* Clinton proposal of 1993.
9. Note, however, that Medicare developed in the 1980s an analogous structure of

225

neocorporatism for both hospital and physician reimbursement: the Prospective
Payment Commission (ProPac) and the Physician Payment Review Commission.
For the origins of this American analogue to corporatism, see Lawrence D.
Brown, "Technocratic Corporatism and Administrative Reform in Medicare,"
Journal of Health Politics, Policy, and Law, Vol. 10, No. 3 (Fall 1985), pp. 579–
99.

CHAPTER 2: HOW WE GOT TO WHERE WE ARE

1. The sketch of American medical politics and policy is drawn from my previous
   work: "Commentary" [on Kenneth R. Wing, "American Health Policy in the
   1980s," *Case Western Reserve Law Review,* Vol. 36, No. 4 (1985–1986), pp. 608–
   85], *Case Western Reserve Law Review,* Vol. 36, No. 4 (1985–1986), pp. 686–92;
   and from a review of Robert G. Evans, *Strained Mercy: The Economics of Cana-*
   dian Health Care (Toronto: Butterworths, 1984), in *Journal of Health Politics,*
   Policy, and Law, Vol. 11, No. 1 (1986), pp. 163–66; expanded version in *Perspec-*
   tives in Biology and Medicine, Vol. 30, No. 4 (1987), pp. 590–96.
2. Edward M. Kennedy, *In Critical Condition: The Crisis in America's Health Care*
   (New York: Simon and Schuster, 1972).
3. The politics of this period are reviewed in Lawrence D. Brown, *Politics and*
   Health Care Organizations: HMOs as Federal Policy (Washington, D.C.: Brook-
   ings, 1984); and T. R. Marmor, *Political Analysis and American Medical Care*
   (New York: Cambridge University Press, 1983).
4. For a varied discussion of these new elements in American medicine, see Jeffrey
   Goldsmith, "Death of a Paradigm: The Challenge of Competition," *Health Affairs,*
   Vol. 3 (Fall 1984), pp. 7–19; Paul Starr, *The Social Transformation of American*
   Medicine (New York: Basic Books, 1984); and T. R. Marmor, Mark Schlesinger,
   and Richard W. Smithey, "A New Look at Nonprofits: Health Care Policy in a
   Competitive Age," *Yale Journal of Regulation,* Vol. 3 (Spring 1986), pp. 313–49
   [Chapter 4 in this book].
5. See, for instance, Henry J. Aaron and William B. Schwartz, *The Painful Prescrip-*
   tion: Rationing Health Care (Washington, D.C.: Brookings, 1983).
6. See Alan C. Enthoven, *Health Plan: The Only Practical Solution to Soaring*
   Health Care Costs (Reading, Mass.: Addison-Wesley, 1980); Clark C. Havighurst,
   "Competition in Health Services: Overview, Issues, and Answers," *Vanderbilt*
   Law Review, Vol. 34 (May 1981), pp. 1115–78; and T. R. Marmor, Richard Boyer,
   and Julie Greenberg, "Medical Care and Procompetitive Reform," *Vanderbilt Law*
   Review, Vol. 34 (May 1981), pp. 1003–28.
7. These ideas are drawn from T. R. Marmor and Jon B. Christianson, *Health Care*
   Policy: A Political Economy Approach (Los Angeles: Sage Publications, 1982).
8. Brian Abel-Smith, *Value for Money in Health Services* (London: Heinemann Educational Books, 1976).
9. For an extended presentation of the politics of medical inflation, see Wing,
   "American Health Policy in the 1980s."

10. For a fuller development of this point, see Wing, "American Health Policy in the 1980s"; T. R. Marmor, D. A. Wittman, and T. C. Heagy, "The Politics of Medical Inflation," in Marmor, *Political Analysis and American Medical Care;* T. R. Marmor and Andrew Dunham, "The Politics of Health Policy Reform: Problems, Origins, Alternatives, and a Possible Prescription" in *Health Care: How to Improve It and Pay for It* (Washington, D.C.: Center for National Policy, 1985), pp. 33–44; and T. R. Marmor and R. Klein, "Cost vs. Care: America's Health Care Dilemma Wrongly Considered," *Health Matrix,* Vol. 4, No. 1 (Spring 1986), pp. 19–24 [Chapter 6 in this book].
11. Wing, "American Health Policy in the 1980s," p. 610.
12. Wing, "American Health Policy in the 1980s," p. 612.
13. Wing, "American Health Policy in the 1980s," p. 612.
14. See T. R. Marmor, review of Eli Ginzberg, *American Medicine: The Power Shift* (Totowa, N.J.: Rowman & Allaheid, 1985), and of Victor Fuchs, *The Health Economy* (Cambridge, Mass.: Harvard University Press, 1986), *American Political Science Review,* Vol. 82 (1988), pp. 633–37.
15. James A. Morone and T. R. Marmor, "Representing Consumer Interests: The Case of American Health Planning," in Marmor, *Political Analysis and American Medical Care.*
16. See note 1.
17. Robert Y. Shapiro and John T. Young, "The Polls: Medical Care in the United States," *Public Opinion Quarterly,* Vol. 50 (1986), pp. 418–28.
18. More recent polls (from 1989) that compared public opinion about health care in the United States, Canada, and the United Kingdom echo these earlier results. Of the Americans polled, 89 percent felt their system needed fundamental change; 42 percent of the Canadians and 69 percent of the British felt the same way about their systems. Nor were Americans any more happy with the care they received. Only 35 percent of those polled indicated satisfaction with the health care services they received, as compared with a satisfaction rate of 6 percent in Canada. See Dennis Hevesi, "Polls Show Discontent with Health Care," *New York Times,* February 15, 1989.
19. Mancur Olson, *The Logic of Collective Action: Public Goods and the Theory of Groups* (Cambridge, Mass.: Harvard University Press, 1965).

CHAPTER 3: MEDICAL CARE CRISES AND THE WELFARE STATE

1. See T. R. Marmor, A. Bridges, and W. L. Hoffman, "Comparative Politics and Health Policies: Notes on Benefits, Costs, Limits," in *Political Analysis and American Medical Care: Essays,* T. R. Marmor, editor (New York: Cambridge University Press, 1983) for a discussion of the uses of cross-national evidence in health policy. More generally, see D. E. Ashford, editor, *Comparing Public Policies: New Concepts and Methods* (Beverly Hills, Calif.: Sage Publications, 1978).
2. See, for example, Robert B. Reich, "Bailout: A Comparative Study in Law and Industrial Structure," *Yale Journal on Regulation* 2 (No. 2, 1985): 163–224.

3. Sweden and Australia in the late 1970s, and later France, Germany, and Canada.

4. New Brunswick, N.J.: Transaction Books, 1981.

5. Organization for Economic Cooperation and Development, *The Welfare State in Crisis: An Account of the Conference on Social Policies in the 1980s* (Paris: OECD, 1981). The conference took place in Paris, October 20–23, 1980.

6. Richard Rose and Guy Peters, *Can Government Go Bankrupt?* (New York: Basic Books, 1978).

7. Rudolf Klein and Michael O'Higgins, "Defusing the Crisis of the Welfare State: A New Interpretation," in *Social Security: Beyond the Rhetoric of Crisis,* T. Marmor and J. Mashaw, editors (Princeton: Princeton University Press, 1988).

8. For further discussion, see David Cameron, "On the Limits of the Public Economy," *Annals of the American Academy of Political and Social Science* 459 (1982), and Manfred Schmidt, "The Welfare State and the Economy in Periods of Economic Crisis," *European Journal of Political Research* 11 (1983): 1–26.

9. Daniel Tarschys, "Curbing Public Expenditure: Current Trends," *Journal of Public Policy* (No. 7, 1985): 23–67.

10. See, for example, Peter G. Peterson, "Social Security: The Coming Crash," *New York Review of Books,* December 2, 1982.

11. John Palmer and Barbara Torrey, "Health Care Financing and Pension Programs," in *Federal Budget Policy in the 1980s,* Gregory Mille and John Palmer, editors (Washington, D.C.: Urban Institute, 1984).

12. See Robert T. Kudrle and Theodore R. Marmor, "The Development of Welfare States in North America," in *The Development of Welfare States in Europe and America,* P. Flora and A. J. Heidenheimer, editors (New Brunswick, N.J.: Transaction Books, 1981), especially pp. 114–16.

13. The celebrated public disputes over Charles Murray's book, *Losing Ground* (New York: Basic Books, 1985) are illustrative. Few such exchanges have addressed Social Security pensions or Medicare, programs that are overwhelmingly more significant fiscally (as Table 3.2 shows) than the whole nest of poverty and public programs.

14. It is true that some critics of public welfare, such as Murray, also emphasize the consequences for work of public assistance rules and regulations.

15. Flora and Heidenheimer, *The Development of Welfare States in Europe and America.*

16. Klein and O'Higgins, "Defusing the Crisis of the Welfare State."

17. Organization for Economic Cooperation and Development, *Social Expenditure: 1960–1981, Problems of Growth and Control* (Paris: OECD, 1985). Klein and O'Higgins are careful to note the limitations as well as the benefits of using this particular data source. While it does make comparable data conveniently available, it has the disadvantage of ending its time series in 1981. Further, by treating the periods 1960–1975 and 1975–1981 as though each were homogeneous, the study may suggest conclusions that would not hold if the focus of analysis were on trends *within* each of these periods. In addition, the particular form of presentation for these data begs the question of whether, in the words of the OECD report, "the passage

of time would probably have seen some automatic moderation as the major social programmes approached maturity" (p. 9). They also note the following additional difficulties with the OECD data. First, social expenditure, defined as spending on education, health care, pensions, and unemployment compensation, ignores spending on means-tested social assistance and also ignores possible substitution effects between different types of programs. Second, the data ignore tax expenditures. And yet, they note, "some of the most significant shifts in public policy, particularly in terms of their distributional effects, have taken the form of tilting the balance between direct and tax spending." Klein and O'Higgins, "Defusing the Crisis of the Welfare State," p. 8.

18. Details of this analysis can be found in Klein and O'Higgins, "Defusing the Crisis of the Welfare State."

19. The income elasticity of social expenditures is defined as the ratio of the growth rate of nominal social expenditures to the growth rate of nominal GDP (Gross Domestic Product). An income elasticity of less than 1.0 indicates that the country's economy grew at a faster rate than its social expenditures. An elasticity of 1.0 indicates that a given percentage increase in economic growth was matched by the same percentage increase in social expenditures.

20. See Francis G. Castles, editor, *The Impact of Parties* (London: Sage, 1982) and Harold L. Wilensky, Gregory M. Luebbert, Susan R. Hahn, and Adrienne M. Jamieson, *Comparative Social Policy* (Berkeley, Institute of International Studies, 1985).

21. Klein and O'Higgins, "Defusing the Crisis of the Welfare State."

22. T. R. Marmor, *The Politics of Medicare* (Chicago: Aldine, 1973).

23. Klein and O'Higgins, "Defusing the Crisis of the Welfare State."

24. Paul Light, *Artful Work: The Politics of Social Security Reform* (New York: Random House, 1985). The exchange in the *New York Review of Books* between Peter J. Peterson ("Social Security: The Coming Crash," December 2, 1982; "The Salvation of Social Security," December 16, 1982; and "A Reply to Critics," March 17, 1986) and Alicia Munnell ("A Calmer Look at Social Security," March 17, 1983) illustrates the way in which long-term specters—that is, twenty-first-century developments—were centrally at issue in the commentary on Social Security's 1982 troubles.

CHAPTER 4: NONPROFIT ORGANIZATIONS AND HEALTH CARE

1. As of 1982, there were 34 investor-owned multihospital systems comprising 773 hospitals, and 139 nonprofit systems comprising 967 hospitals (up from 121 nonprofit systems in 1978). Of the almost 7,000 acute-care hospitals in the United States, 11 percent are proprietary and another 4 percent are managed by proprietary organizations. Nonprofit hospitals account for approximately 50 percent of the total. The remainder are operated by federal, state, and local governments. See Gray (1985) for a review of the growth of nonprofit and proprietary hospital systems and recent activity in institutions other than hospitals.

2. In the event, Baxter Travenol won the battle for American Hospital Supply, out-bidding HCA to produce a huge $4 billion conglomerate. Had HCA succeeded, the result would have been the largest U.S. health care firm, a vertically integrated conglomerate with an estimated $7.6 billion in annual revenues (Waldholz 1985, 3; Koten & Waldholz 1985, 2; Koten 1985, 2).

3. This is a major trend among big-city voluntary hospitals. Its extent is evident from the incorporation of Voluntary Hospitals of America, formed by 62 voluntary hos-pitals. Its subsidiary activities, all of which are for-profit, extend to management services, physician recruitment, outpatient services, supply services, financing, and insurance.

4. One example is the debate in the *New England Journal of Medicine* over the propriety of proprietary agencies treating end-stage renal disease (Lowrie & Ham-pers 1982; Relman & Rennie 1980; Lowrie 1981; Gardner 1981).

5. American Medicorp International, Preferred Provider Organization, Hospital Cor-poration of America, Diagnosis-Related Group, and Voluntary Hospitals of Amer-ica.

6. The clash of views is really quite stark. Compare the following examples: "Non-profit hospitals may be operationally inefficient compared to their for-profit coun-terparts. Moreover the nonprofit form may have played a key role in leading to both wasteful overcapacity of medical facilities in some areas and slow response to demand in others, while promoting the development of extremely costly and not truly justified 'high technology' health care" (Clark 1980, 1417–18). Referring to the growth of proprietary organizations in health, Relman (1980) states: "The private health care industry can be expected to ignore relatively inefficient and unprofitable services, regardless of medical or social need. The result is likely to exacerbate present problems with excessive fragmentation of care, overspecializa-tion, and overemphasis on expensive technology" (p. 969). Relman (1983) later claimed, "Judged not as businesses but as hospitals, which are supposed to serve the public interest, they [investor-owned chain hospitals] have been less cost-effective than their not-for-profit counterparts" (p. 372).

　　The American College of Hospital Administrators (now American College of Hospital *Executives*) forecast that 60 percent of all hospitals will be investor owned by 1995 ("Health Care" 1984, 2).

7. The nonprofit has traditionally been the protector of consumers or purchasers of services from "contract failure." By virtue of its distribution prohibition, the non-profit protects the buyer against the misdelivery of services he cannot monitor or understand (Hansmann 1980). Given that, in the case of medical care, this protec-tive role was vested in the doctor as the patient's agent, the traditional role of the nonprofit was really less important.

8. The importance of nonmonetary incentives in medical care has led Evans to define the "not-only-for-profit sector." This refers to individuals and firms "in which a legal claimant to profits is well-defined, but profits represent only one among sev-eral competing objectives of the firm's ownership and management" (1984, 127).

9. The for-profit health care provider usually takes on the familiar corporate form. In

particular, the company is owned by its stockholders and managed by a board of directors elected by the stockholders. Capital is raised through the sale of equity and the issuance of debt. Any net earnings are distributed in the form of dividends to the stockholders or retained and reinvested by the corporation, rendering the stock more valuable.

The nonprofit corporation, in comparison, does not issue equity. Capital is raised by collection of donations and issuance of debt. A nonprofit may accrue net earnings, but no dividends are paid. Any net earnings must be retained by the corporation. (A commercial nonprofit organization must make a profit to survive, especially in medical care. The distinction between nonprofit and for-profit enterprise rests largely on what is termed the nondistribution constraint—that is, profits cannot be distributed to individuals.) The corporation is managed most often by a board of directors, either elected by the membership (which can include either donors or beneficiaries) or self-perpetuating. Thus, unlike the for-profit corporation, there is no formal connection between an individual's financial interest in the venture and the power to select and control management. Furthermore, given the prohibition against equity sales and the often slow process of raising funds through donation drives, the nonprofits in health are at a relative disadvantage in terms of their ability to generate capital funds.

Some, but not all, nonprofit corporations are charities under Section 501(c)3 of the federal tax law, I.R.C. 501(c)3 (1982). All nonprofit hospitals, for instance, are characterized as charities, whereas a nonprofit insurance company or testing laboratory would not be a charity. The charity status is important because donations to charitable organizations are tax deductible to the donor, thus conferring a significant federal subsidy on nonprofit charities that receive contributions. State and federal tax laws also define a category of nonprofits, broader than the category of charities, that are exempt from corporate income, sales, and other taxes.

Hansmann has developed a useful scheme for describing differences among nonprofits, which identifies two characteristics: the source of income and the form of management or control. The "donative nonprofit" relies primarily on donation income; the "commercial nonprofit" derives its income primarily from the sales of goods or services to paying consumers; the "mutual nonprofit" is run by a board selected by the donor or consumer members; and the "entrepreneurial nonprofit" is managed by a self-selected board. The dominant form of nonprofit in the health care industry is the entrepreneurial/commercial nonprofit. Nonprofit hospitals, although they qualify as charities, receive the great bulk of their income from sale of services. Donations to a nursing home are more rare (Hansmann 1980).

The third set of actors in health care are the public providers. Cities, counties, states, and the federal government all operate hospital and health facilities of various kinds. The capital funds are tax dollars, and the management is under the formal control of the sponsoring government.

10. One view suggests that American medicine became more mercenary in 1920 with a change of control in American medicine to a new group of leaders. Their purpose was to improve their economic position and protect their freedom from social

or governmental controls. Nielsen asserts that because the individual states worked closely with and patterned their licensing statutes on those suggested by the American Medical Association (AMA) and state medical societies, the AMA was largely responsible for a 30 percent decline in the number of proprietary medical schools and a 50 percent decrease in the number of medical graduates (Nielsen 1979, 106).

11. For a review of AMA resistance to various other forms of health insurance as well as the "corporate" practice of medicine, see Starr (1982, 295ff.) and Nielsen (1979, 105–16).

12. In the case of *Associated Hospital Service Inc.* v. *City of Milwaukee* (1961), for example, the court concluded that the legislature had the right to grant nonprofit status to the Blue Cross plan specifically because it was closely associated with nonprofit hospitals. (The American Hospital Association owned the name "Blue Cross of America" until 1972.)

13. About half the states refused to grant the plans tax-exempt status. As of 1978 the 20 states that granted exempt status were Arizona, Arkansas, California, Connecticut, Georgia, Idaho, Illinois, Kentucky, Louisiana, Maine, Massachusetts, Michigan, New Jersey, New York, North Carolina, Ohio, Oklahoma, Vermont, West Virginia, and Wisconsin (Law 1974, 9n37).

   According to Law (1974): "Special corporate status and exemption from federal and state taxes seem to be based on a concept of social reform and utility rather than on any particular concrete characteristics of the Blue Cross plans. Neither the legislative history nor cases involving the validity of the tax-exempt status provide much insight into the justification for the favored status of hospital service plans over commercial hospital insurers. State tax exemption has been challenged by tax collectors in five states. In all but one, the courts held that the Blue Cross was not entitled to exemption from payment of state taxes, even though it has been characterized as charitable or benevolent by the legislature" (p. 9).

   Blue Cross plans are exempt from federal income tax under I.R.C. 501(c)4. A 501(c)4 organization is exempt from federal income tax, but contributions to such an organization are not tax deductible by the contributor (Law 1974, 9–10).

14. Coverage was rarely offered on a sliding scale or discounted in any other fashion for low-income subscribers (Starr 1982, 309; Feldstein 1978, 183; Law 1974, 12).

15. Between 1945 and 1960, the number of beds in short-term public hospitals increased from approximately 133,000 to 156,000. Between 1949 and 1959 the number of beds in public psychiatric hospitals increased from 596,000 to 672,000, and from 1954 to 1973 the number of beds in public nursing homes increased from 27,000 to 106,000 (Schlesinger 1984, 76–77).

16. Although the short-term growth of proprietary providers occurred for all these services, for some, such as hospitalization, the growth of for-profit facilities has been much more pronounced over the long term (Sloan & Vraciu 1983).

17. The federal government passed the National Health Planning and Resources Development Act of 1974, 42 U.S.C. par. 300e-4, 300k et seq. (1976), which authorized a system of local health planning organizations or health systems agencies

(HSAs) to be dominated by consumers, to be designed to cut the costs of medical care, and to guarantee the quality of and improve the access to that care. The restraining effects of these HSAs, however, were modest (Morone & Marmor 1983; Starr 1982, 416). Certificate of Need (CON) programs, which required state (and HSA) approval of construction, and large capital programs planned by medical institutions were other cost-control devices (Starr 1982, 398). Other regulatory attempts to control medical costs have included requirements for prior authorization, restrictions on capital expenditures, and reductions in the number of hospital beds (E. Brown 1983, 936–37). See also Marmor, Wittman, & Heagy (1983); Enthoven (1980); Marmor & Dunham (1985); and Brown (1986).

An effort to control the quality as well as the cost of medical care was the Professional Standards Review Organizations (PSROs), which functioned "by reviewing admissions to a health care facility, certifying the necessity for continuing treatment in an in-patient facility, reviewing other extended or costly treatment, conducting medical evaluation studies, regularly reviewing facility, practitioner, and health care profiles of care and reviewing facility and practitioner records as applicable to a particular review process" (Raffel 1980, 282).

Increasingly numerous as an alternative are HMOs. Patients must pay a flat annual sum, and they directly receive a wide array of medical services. The HMO must provide services within a fixed budget determined by the number of providers. In the 1980s, the federal government attempted to control costs by using DRGs, which establish price limitations on a variety of hospital services (Morone & Dunham 1985; Comptroller General 1980, 34–62; Brown 1985).

18. This growth should be interpreted with caution. In simple terms, doubling market share in any industry from 5 to 10 percent is easier than increasing that share from 10 to 20 percent or from 20 to 40 percent. The base of HMO enrollment was quite low in the mid-1970s, and the doubling of its clientele from that base did not necessarily foreshadow similar rates of growth on the higher base. Second, what counts as an HMO has, over time, been defined more loosely: it also includes groups of physicians coordinated under the prepayment rubric of IPAs (individual practice associations). Third, as HMOs have grown, they have increasingly come to be owned by other firms in the health industry: Blue Cross, Blue Shield, commercial health insurance firms such as Prudential, and some for-profit hospital chains. These changes in corporate governance make the character of the HMO population quite different from the model organization envisioned in the HMO act of 1973. Finally, it hardly needs pointing out that it is the financial incentives of prepaid group practice, not the legal category of HMOs, that explain most of the cost-restraining effects associated in the literature with HMOs. Luft (1981) rightly cautions that most of the cost-saving effects arise from more restrained use of hospitalization, some of which in turn is explained by the healthier populations who joined the earlier groups. Over time, the rate of increase in HMO costs have paralleled medical inflation, thus suggesting that the effects of HMO growth on inflation control have been exaggerated (L. Brown 1983).

19. Most health insurance plans, for instance, do not cover the costs of experimental

procedures. It is only when such care is provided on a sufficiently widespread basis that it is covered and thus affordable for most individuals.

20. About half of these are reviewed and summarized in Bishop (1980). Since that review was published, additional research has been completed by Koetting (1980), Frech & Ginsburg (1981), Caswell & Cleverly (1983), and Schlenker & Shaughnessy (1984).

21. Related research supports this pattern. For-profit providers appear to have lower costs in the provision of laboratory services (Danzon 1982) and health insurance (Frech 1976), but to have equal or higher costs for renal dialysis centers (Held & Pauly 1982) and health maintenance organizations (Schlesinger, Blumenthal, & Schlesinger 1986).

22. Studies comparing for-profit and nonprofit nursing homes have concluded variously that for-profit institutions have quality that is equal to nonprofit homes (Holmberg & Anderson 1968; Ullman 1983), less than nonprofit facilities (Koetting 1980), or equal in some dimensions but less in others (Riportella-Mueller & Slesinger 1982; Weisbrod & Schlesinger 1981).

23. Critics argue that proprietary hospitals engage in two forms of cream skimming: those involving services and those involving the selection of patients. According to this view, they skimp on expensive and underutilized services and exclude patients with complex illnesses who are uninsured or covered by Medicaid and cannot pay their full charges (Steinwald & Neuhauser 1970, 832).

24. Thus hospitals use revenues from full-paying patients to subsidize the Medicare and Medicaid patients. Even for-profit hospitals accept a substantial discount on the cost of care (Sloan & Vraciu 1983, 33).

25. The differences between predicted and current costs of "transferred" patients are small, on the border of 2 to 4 percent. Each individual difference is statistically insignificant, and the cost difference between patients in public nursing homes and those in for-profit homes is opposite to that predicted. Nonetheless, 11 of the 12 signs are as one would predict if for-profit facilities did screen patients on the basis of costs. This pattern would occur by chance with a probability of less than 0.003.

26. The figures represent 7.5 percent of GNP in 1970 (Table 4.3) and about 11 percent in 1983.

27. To use these differences to further social ends, however, requires a fairly sophisticated and complicated set of policies. Past ownership-based interventions have often been crude and, as a result, have met with mixed success. When, for example, California adopted a prepaid system of care for its Medi-Cal enrollees, policymakers were concerned that prepayment would create incentives to cut quality of care. To mitigate these incentives, they required that all participating prepaid plans be organized under nonprofit auspices, on the theory that this would prevent providers from having a monetary incentive to reduce quality. This strategy was circumvented by entrepreneurs who established a set of nonprofit dummy corporations that effectively funneled profits to subsidiaries, creating essentially the same

incentives as if the plans had been organized as proprietary corporations (Goldberg 1975).

28. Surely the potential for growth exists. As Evans notes about the for-profit testing lab: "The strong stimulus to 'more' which is a consequence of for-profit motivation justifies serious concern. Unnecessary testing is pure waste of resources. But for-profit organization does not, cannot, recognize unnecessary testing as an intellectual concept. Sales are their own justification" (1984, 321).

29. As Morone has observed, "For-profit chains scramble the traditional discourse over American health policy by setting the principles of free enterprise and physician autonomy into tension" (1985, 4). Actually, this tension has long been present in American health care, but it took large and powerful corporations to adopt the profession's ideology with a vengeance.

30. Generally, both public and private hospitals have a duty to accept all patients who require emergency care. That duty does not extend, however, to nonemergency situations (Marsh 1985, 162; *Stanford Law Review* 1962; Grady 1986).

CHAPTER 5: CUTTING WASTE BY MAKING RULES

1. *See* Katharine R. Levit et al., *National Health Expenditures, 1990,* Health Care Financing Rev., Fall 1991, at 29, 30.

2. *See* Bureau of Census, U.S. Dep't of Commerce, Statistical Abstract of the United States 1990, at 92 (110th ed. 1990).

3. *See id.*

4. The topic of rationing first drew widespread attention with the publication of Aaron and Schwartz's pioneering comparative study of the scale and distribution of therapeutic procedures under Britain's National Health Service and America's health care system. *See* Henry J. Aaron and William B. Schwartz, The Painful Prescription: Rationing Hospital Care (1984). Their argument, that British-style rationing decisions will inevitably need to be made in this country, has subsequently been elaborated upon. *See* William B. Schwartz, *The Inevitable Failure of Current Cost-Containment Strategies: Why They Can Parade Only Temporary Relief,* 257 JAMA 220 (1987). For a critical analysis, see Theodore Marmor & Rudolf Klein, *Costs Versus Care: America's Health Care Dilemma Wrongly Considered,* 4 Health Matrix 19 (1986).

   A second wave of popular attention to rationing accompanied Oregon's controversial and widely noted proposal to alter the list of reimbursable services under the Medicaid program. For an evenhanded description of that program, under which reimbursement decisions would be guided by "cost-effectiveness" considerations, see Daniel M. Fox and Howard M. Leichter, *Rationing Health Care in Oregon: The New Accountability,* Health Aff., Summer 1991, at 7; for an illuminating discussion of the politics surrounding the plan, see Lawrence D. Brown, *The National Politics of Oregon's Rationing Plan,* Health Aff., Summer 1991, at 28; for an analysis of the ethical issues it raises, see Norman Daniels, *Is the Ore-*

gon Rationing Plan Fair?, 265 JAMA 2232 (1991); and for a particularly critical review of the plan as an effort to limit services to the poor, see Bruce C. Vladeck, *Unhealthy Rations,* Am. Prospect, Summer 1991, at 101.

5. *See* Theodore R. Marmor & Jan Blustein, *Introduction to Rationing,* 140 U. Pa. L. Rev. 1539 (1992).

6. A reader of the popular press might well conclude that one-quarter to one-half of present medical practice is "pure waste," benefiting no one. For example, according to a *New York Times* op-ed piece of a few years ago: "The evidence is now overwhelming that at least twenty-five percent of the money that Americans spend on health care is wasted. . . . There is a growing consensus that half the coronary bypasses, most Caesarean sections and a significant proportion of many other procedures . . . are unnecessary. A former editor of [*JAMA*] is convinced that more than half of the 40 million medical tests performed each year 'do not really contribute to a patient's diagnosis or therapy.'" Joseph A. Califano, Jr., *Billions Blown on Health,* N.Y. Times, Apr. 12, 1989, at A25.

7. *See James S. Todd, M.D.: Only Parameters Will Give MDs Needed Flexibility,* Am. Med. News, Jan. 6, 1989, at 23, 23 [hereinafter *Todd Interview*] (interview with AMA Senior Deputy Executive Vice President).

8. *See* Agency for Health Care Policy and Research, U.S. Dep't of Health and Human Servs., Program Note: Clinical Guideline Development (1990) [hereinafter AHCPR, Program Note].

9. *See* Mark R. Chassin, *Standards of Care in Medicine,* 25 Inquiry 437, 437 (1988).

10. This chapter does not address techniques such as "physician profiling," whereby payers examine physicians' *patterns* of care in order to detect tendencies toward inappropriate or wasteful use of services. *See* Robert W. Dubois, *Reducing Unnecessary Care: Different Approaches to the "Big Ticket" and the "Little Ticket" Items,* J. Ambulatory Care Mgmt., October 1991, at 30; Milt Freudenheim, *Software Controls on Health Costs,* N.Y. Times, Feb. 18, 1992, at D2. Many of our comments apply equally well to these newer approaches, however.

11. Those falling into this last category are often said to be "not cost-effective," but this term is all too often used imprecisely. In the medical literature "cost-effective" has been variously taken to be synonymous with "cost-saving," "effective," and "having an additional benefit worth the cost." *See* Peter Doubilet et al., *Use and Misuse of the Term 'Cost-Effective' in Medicine,* 314 New Eng. J. Med. 253, 253–54 (1986).

12. *See* Robert H. Brook & Kathleen N. Lohr, *Will We Need to Ration Effective Health Care?,* Issues Sci. & Tech., Fall 1986, at 68, 72.

13. *See* Marcia Angell, *Cost Containment and the Physician,* 254 JAMA 1203, 1204 (1985).

14. *See Todd Interview, supra* note 7, at 23.

15. The rules to which we refer emanate from the Health Care Financing Administration. Although the precise content of these rules, as developed and enforced by HCFA's financial intermediaries, is confidential, a general description may be found

in Health Care Fin. Admin., Medical Carriers Manual § 7500ff. (HCFA Pub. 14) (1990).

16. *Are Guidelines, Standards or Parameters Having an Impact on the Way You Practice Medicine, and How?*, Am. Med. News, Jan 6, 1989, at 34 (interviewing a private practitioner in St. Louis).

17. Glenn Kramon, *Taking a Scalpel to Health Costs*, N.Y. Times, Jan. 8, 1989, § 3, at 1, 9 (quoting the vice president of a cost-management company).

18. Ivan Illich, Medical Nemesis (1976).

19. *Id.* at 44.

20. *Id.* at 114 (emphasis omitted).

21. Edmund Faltermeyer, *Medical Care's Next Revolution*, Fortune, Oct. 10, 1988, at 126.

22. *See* Arnold M. Epstein, *The Outcomes Movement—Will It Get Us Where We Want to Go?*, 323 New Eng. J. Med. 266, 268 (1990); David M. Eddy & John Billings, *The Quality of Medical Evidence: Implications for Quality of Care*, Health Aff., Spring 1988, at 19, 28–29.

23. *See* Eddy & Billings, *supra* note 22, at 28.

24. These other methodologies, often subsumed under the rubric of "observational epidemiology," are clearly elucidated in J. Mark Ellwood, Causal Relationships in Medicine: A Practical System of Critical Appraisal (1988). For a nontechnical account of the pitfalls of such studies, see Max Michael et al., Biomedical Bestiary: An Epidemiologic Guide to Flaws and Fallacies in the Medical Literature (1984).

25. *See* Epstein, *supra* note 22, at 268; Eddy & Billings, *supra* note 22, at 20. We do not wish to create the impression that little of value is known about effectiveness in clinical medicine. As one of our readers, Dr. Colin Dayan, has pointed out, there are numerous cases in which researchers have conclusively demonstrated the effectiveness (or lack thereof) of particular interventions. These cases notwithstanding, no one doubts that much remains to be learned about the utility of present practices.

26. *See* Robert W. Dubois & Robert H. Brook, *Assessing Clinical Decision Making: Is the Ideal System Feasible?*, 25 Inquiry 59, 63 (1988); Eddy & Billings, *supra* note 22, at 24.

27. For a discussion of the specific methods used to develop the appropriateness ratings, see Rolla E. Park et al., *Physician Ratings of Appropriate Indications for Six Medical and Surgical Procedures*, 76 Am. J. Pub. Health 766 (1986).

28. *See id.* at 767.

29. *See id.* at 768–69.

30. *See id.* at 767.

31. *See* Harris Meyer, *Payers to Use Protocols to Assess Treatment Plans*, Am. Med. News, Dec. 9, 1988, at 1, 62–63. Actual refusal rates have increased, as early versions of the software have been replaced by more sophisticated programs. *See* telephone Interview with Dr. Robert DeBois, Senior Vice President of Value Health Sciences (Mar. 2, 1992); *infra* note 78 and accompanying text.

32. *See* Epstein, *supra* note 22, at 266.
33. These differences in perception have taken several forms. Some participants have emphasized the movement's potential to cut costs, see Brook & Lohr, *supra* note 12, at 68; Califano, *supra* note 6, at A25; Faltermeyer, *supra* note 21, at 126; others have highlighted its promise of harnessing scientific knowledge to enhance the quality of medical care, see Agency for Health Care Policy and Research, U.S. Dep't of Health and Human Servs., Research Activities 4 (1992) [hereinafter AHCPR, Research]; William L. Roper et al., *Effectiveness in Health Care: An Initiative to Evaluate and Improve Medical Practice,* 319 New Eng. J. Med. 1197, 1197 (1988). Some members have embraced the idea of using rules to audit physicians' practice choices, see *supra* notes 27–32 and accompanying text. Others, reluctant to promote "cookbook medicine," and believing that physicians will respond to education about "appropriate" practices, appear to prefer that adherence to guidelines be kept voluntary. *See* AHCPR, Research, *supra,* at 5. *See also infra* note 80. This preference may be optimistic in light of previous studies showing that physician practice choices are relatively resistant to the "practice suggestions" of experts. *See, e.g.,* Jacqueline Kosecoff et al., *Effects of the National Institutes of Health Consensus Development Program on Physician Practice,* 258 JAMA 2708, 2712 (1987) (finding that consensus development conferences produced little change in patient care); Jonathan Lomas et al., *Do Practice Guidelines Guide Practice? The Effect of Consensus Statements on the Practice of Physicians,* 321 New Eng. J. Med. 1306, 1310 (1989) (concluding that while practice guidelines may affect "the perceptions of physicians," they alone are insufficient to alter physicians' behavior). Other incentives may be needed to modify practice patterns. The range of alternatives is canvassed in John M. Eisenberg, *Physician Utilization: The State of Research about Physicians' Practice Patterns,* 23 Med. Care 461, 467–70 (1988).

    Despite these differences in perception, it is undeniable that much of the enthusiasm (and funding) behind the outcomes movement has been driven by the perception that it will slow the rising cost of medical care expenditures, and it is clear that many of the key participants view the development of a link between "appropriate" practices and reimbursement as a foregone conclusion. *See infra* notes 40–42 and accompanying text. In this chapter we explore the implications of implementing such a policy.
34. Paul M. Ellwood, *Shattuck Lecture—Outcomes Management: A Technology of Patient Experience,* 318 New Eng. J. Med. 1549, 1551 (1988).
35. Arnold S. Relman, *Assessment and Accountability: The Third Revolution in Health Care,* 319 New Eng. J. Med. 1220 (1988).
36. *See* Roper et al., *supra* note 33, at 1197.
37 AHCPR, Program Note, *supra* note 8, at 6 (quoting the Legislative Summary to the Omnibus Budget and Reconciliation Act of 1989). Although the AHCPR has been the beneficiary of congressional enthusiasm for medical care cost savings, the Agency's leaders have recently become eager to avoid disappointment, disclaiming a connection between guideline development and cost containment. As the Agency

released the first of its guidelines this spring, its director, Dr. J. Jarrett Clinton, remarked that "there are those in Congress who hoped, and still hope, that this effort would be a cost-savings device, but it has limited use for this purpose. . . . This is not about cost-cutting, but about getting the best value per dollar spent in the long run. In some cases, for instance, the guidelines may result in spending more money on some things. Warren E. Leary, *More Advice for Doctors: U.S. Guides on Treatments,* N.Y. Times, Apr. 15, 1992, at C14. Despite its position in the forefront of the outcomes movement, then, the Agency's perception of the movement's direction may be at odds with that of some of the movement's members and supporters, including some members of Congress, the insurance industry, the business community, and some academic researchers.

38. *See House Subcommittee Votes Level Funding for AHCPR and HCFA: Senate Likely to Increase Support for AHCPR,* HSR Reports (Association for Health Services Research, Washington, D.C.), June 1991, at 1, 5.

39. *See* Epstein, *supra* note 22, at 266.

40. For example, Blue Cross and Blue Shield executive Bernard T. Tresnowski, when asked about the practice parameters approach, responded: "'Right on!'" *See* Faltermeyer, *supra* note 21, at 132. "With better data," it is believed, "business could effectively challenge proposed treatments." *Id.* at 126.

41. See Report of the Board of Trustees of the American Medical Association, Practice Parameters 4 (1990) [hereinafter AMA Trustees' Report] (unpublished report, on file with authors).

42. Sharon McIlrath, *AMA, Rand Corp. Plan for Joint Development of Practice Guidelines,* Am. Med. News, Oct. 28, 1988, at 2.

43. *Todd Interview, supra* note 7, at 25.

44. For an analysis by a physician and leading researcher in the outcomes movement stressing the advantages of practice parameters, see Robert H. Brook, *Practice Guidelines and Practicing Medicine: Are They Compatible?,* 262 JAMA 3027, 3030 (1989).

45. The relationship between practice guidelines and malpractice liability remains a point of considerable controversy among commentators, *See infra* notes 67–70 and accompanying text.

46. *See* telephone Interview with Robert Isquith, Chief of Public Affairs, AHCPR (Mar. 3, 1992); telephone Interview with Stephen H. King, M.D, Chief Medical Officer, AHCPR (July 15, 1991).

47. See Steffie Woolhandler and David U. Himmelstein, *The Deteriorating Administrative Efficiency of the U.S. Health Care System,* 324 New Eng. J. Med. 1253, 1254–55 (1991).

48. *See* Gerald W. Grumet, *Health Care Rationing through Inconvenience: The Third Party's Secret Weapon,* 321 New Eng. J. Med. 607, 608 (1988).

49. Faltermeyer, *supra* note 21 (quoting Dr. Paul M. Ellwood).

50. This option is discussed in detail in Brook, *supra* note 44, at 3029. The idea behind "of unverified effectiveness" would seem to correspond with the RAND categorization "equivocal." *See* Park et al., *supra* note 27, at 767. Much of the popular

commentary following the release of the RAND results, see *supra* text accompanying notes 31–34, conveyed the impression that half of all coronary bypass surgery had been discovered to be medically unnecessary. *See supra* note 6. Yet the RAND group's findings categorized 14 percent of such surgeries as "inappropriate," while 30 percent were classed as "equivocal"; it would thus appear that procedures falling under both of these headings were lumped together in arriving at the "one-half" estimate. *See* Constance M. Winslow et al., *The Appropriateness of Performing Coronary Artery Bypass Surgery,* 260 JAMA 505, 509 (1988). We contend that, from the perspective of health care policymaking, "inappropriate" and "equivocal" procedures are quite different, and that programs aimed at cutting these two distinct types of "waste" would for that reason meet quite different fates.

51. Meyer, *supra* note 31, at 63.

52. McIlrath, *supra* note 42, at 41.

53. A fascinating analysis of these developments can be found in David J. Rothman, Strangers at the Bedside: A History of How Law and Bioethics Transformed Medical Decision Making (1991).

54 *See generally* Daniel Callahan, Setting Limits: Medical Goals in an Aging Society (1987) (contending that medical care should be rationed based on age); Norman Daniels, Am I My Parents' Keeper? An Essay on Justice Between the Young and the Old (1988) (examining the competing claims of the young and the elderly to medical resources); Norman Daniels, Just Health Care (1985) (arguing that a principle of equality of opportunity should guide distribution of health care services); A. A. Scitovsky and A. M. Capron, *Medical Care at the End of Life: The Interaction of Economics and Ethics,* 7 Ann. Rev. Pub. Health 59 (1986) (analyzing the ethical implications of devoting a disproportionate amount of medical resources to the aged); Anne A. Scitovsky, *"The High Cost of Dying": What Do the Data Show?,* 62 Milbank Memorial Fund Q. 591 (1984) (same).

55. *See, e.g., In re* Conroy, 486 A.2d 1209, 1220 (N.J. 1985) (citing *President's Commission for the Study of Ethical Problems,* in Medicine and Biomedical and Behavioral Research, Deciding to Forgo Life-Sustaining Treatment 23 (1983) in an analysis of the question of when life-sustaining treatment may be withdrawn from legally incompetent patients).

56. *See* Callahan, *supra* note 54.

57. *See* Daniel Callahan, *Rethinking Health Care for the Aged,* N.Y. Times, Sept. 25, 1987, at A39.

58. *See Health Debate Rages over Rationing by Age,* AARP News Bull., June 1988, at 1 (quoting comments made by Nat Hentoff at a debate sponsored by the National Council on Aging).

59. *See* David M. Eddy et al., *The Value of Mammography Screening in Women under Age 50 Years,* 259 JAMA 1512, 1512–19 (1988). For completeness we should note that the case is more complicated than suggested above. Though the point remains that mammography is of relatively low benefit to young women, some

significant health costs, such as the risk of a false positive test, are not mentioned. For example, of one hundred women undergoing mammography, one will be referred for a breast biopsy to investigate a radiologic abnormality that turns out not to be cancer. This raises the question of whether the health and social costs of tens of thousands of unnecessary surgeries each year outweigh the benefit of a few hundred lives saved. For an analysis that emphasizes these costs, see John C. Bailar, *Mammography before Age 50 Years?*, 259 JAMA 1548–49 (1988).

60. *See* Annetta Miller et al., *Can You Afford to Get Sick?*, Newsweek, Jan. 30, 1989, at 47.

61. *See* Robert H. Blank, Rationing Medicine 41 (1988).

62. Cost-benefit analysis is but one form of utilitarian program analysis. Other methods include cost-utility analysis and cost-effectiveness analysis. The application of these techniques to medical care is thoroughly discussed in Michael F. Drummond et al., Methods for the Economic Evaluation of Health Care Programmes 74–167 (1987). In this section we refer to cost-benefit analysis, but many of our comments apply as well to the other related forms of analysis.

63. The theoretical difficulties involved are discussed in some detail in Blank, *supra* note 61, at 115–16. An actual illustration arose in Oregon, where the rigorous application of cost-benefit techniques led to a rank ordering of therapies in which the treatment of crooked teeth was placed above therapy for early Hodgkin's disease, and treatment for thumb-sucking was put above hospitalization of a starving child. *See* Fox & Leichter, *supra* note 4, at 22. Although this original list was subsequently reordered, the initial result exposes the conceptual and empirical weakness of utilitarian program analysis as it applies to medical care.

64. *See* Jane Gross, *Turning Disease into Political Cause: First AIDS, and Now Breast Cancer,* N.Y. Times, Jan. 7, 1991, at A12.

65. *See* Fox & Leichter, *supra* note 4, at 23.

66. *See* Robert J. Blendon, *The Public's View of the Future of Health Care,* 259 JAMA 3587, 3590 (1987).

67. *See* Blank, *Supra* note 61, at 137.

68. *See* Harris Meyer, *Managed Care: HMOs Tighten Their Belts, Look to Hybrid Plans and Brighter Future,* Am. Med. News, Jan. 6, 1989, at 12.

69. *See* Troyen A. Brennan, *Practice Guidelines and Malpractice Litigation: Collision or Cohesion?,* 16 J. Health Pol. Pol'y & L. 67, 68; *see also* Mark A. Hall, *The Malpractice Standard under Health Care Cost Containment,* 17 L. Med. & Health Care 347, 353 (1984) (arguing that the "law is fully capable . . . of recognizing the . . . emergence of cost incentives").

70. E. Haavi Morreim, *Stratified Scarcity: Redefining the Standard of Care,* 17 L. Med. & Health Care 356 (1989).

71. *See* Leighton Ku and Dena Fisher, *The Attitudes of Physicians toward Health Care Cost-Containment Policies,* 25 Health Services Res. 25 (1990).

72. *See, e.g.,* Martin I. Broder, *The Impact of Cost Containment on Clinical Care* (Mar. 16–17, 1987), *in* The Health Care Cost Containment Movement: A Reconsid-

eration 9 (report of a conference sponsored by Medicine in the Public Interest, 1988) (arguing that cost-containment programs have had a "disturbing" impact on patient care).

73. Norman G. Levinsky, *The Doctor's Master,* 311 New Eng. J. Med. 1573 (1984).

74. The extent to which such rules can lead to bitterness, cynicism, and professional disengagement is well illustrated in a physician's report of his final 18 hospital visits to an 84-year-old woman dying of lung cancer, visits deemed to be "medically unnecessary." *See* Kenneth M. Prager, *Medicare Meddling,* N.Y. Times, Sept. 12, 1988, at A21.

75. *See* Mark R. Chassin et al., *Does Inappropriate Use Explain Geographic Variations in the Use of Health Care Services? A Study of Three Procedures,* 258 JAMA 2533, 2535 (1987).

76. *See* Epstein, *supra* note 22, at 268.

77. *See* Meyer, *supra* note 31, at 63.

78. *See* Blue Cross and Blue Shield Association, *Preauthorization Review System Finds More than 10 Percent of Medical Procedures Inappropriate,* 8 Med. Benefits 3, 3 (1991). In this case, inappropriate rates varied substantially by procedure, with 27 percent of the proposed tonsillectomies judged to be inappropriate, but none of the proposed heart bypass surgeries or carotid endarterectomies so rated. *See id.* The finding of no inappropriate operations of the 181 bypass procedures is particularly striking in view of the voluminous commentary about the magnitude of "waste" in this category.

79. Other organizations are actively engaged in developing guidelines. For example, many of the medical specialty societies have begun working on parameter development, and by October 1990 had reportedly constructed some 1,000 different guidelines. *See* AMA Trustees' Report, *supra* note 41, at 2. While this work signals enthusiasm for the parameters approach, it also raises the question of how to coordinate the efforts of those involved in the movement to enhance appropriateness and cut waste.

80. *See* Agency for Health Care Policy and Research, U.S. Dep't of Health and Human Services, AHCPR Pub. No. 91-0004, Report to Congress: Progress of Research on Outcomes of Health Care Services and Procedures 13–14 (1991) (discussing the dissemination of information about new technologies and ineffective practices). Policymakers at the agency are working to develop methods to effect change via parameter dissemination, see *id.,* since they are aware of prior studies showing that the practices of physicians are relatively resistant to the "suggestions" of experts, see *supra* note 33.

81. If rulemaking is linked to reimbursement, rules will have to be adopted by many or all payers to achieve widespread savings.

82. *See* Schwartz, *supra* note 4, at 220. It is worth stopping to consider the magnitude of potential economic gains even under the most generous assumptions. If we assume that rulemaking and waste cutting could be implemented for all medical practices over a one-year period (i.e., with 11 percent of present costs instantaneously eliminated), at the end of a decade our health expenditures would total

over 175 percent of real current expenditures, assuming that a 7 percent real inflation rate prevails. If we did not adopt the plan to cut waste, our medical costs at
the end of a decade would be nearly 200 percent of their real present level, again
assuming that inflation continued unabated. If the program to cut waste were
adopted more gradually, the difference between the economic outcomes under the
two scenarios would narrow accordingly.

83. *See generally* Anthony Downs, *Up and Down with Ecology—the "Issue Attention
Cycle,"* 28 Pub. Interest 39, 39 (1972) (noting that "American public attention
rarely remains sharply focused upon any one domestic issue for very long").

84. J. Jarrett Clinton, address to the tenth anniversary meeting of the Association for
Health Services Research (July 1, 1991).

85. *See* Theodore R. Marmor, *American Health Politics 1970 to the Present: Some
Comments,* Q. Rev. Econ. & Bus., Winter 1990, at 32, 32–34.

86. *See* A. J. Culyer, *Cost Containment in Europe, in* Organisation for Economic Cooperation and Development, Health Care Systems in Transition: The Search for
Efficiency 29, 30 (1990).

87. An excellent technical account of these issues can be found in Robert G. Evans,
Strained Mercy: The Economics of Canadian Health Care (1984). For a more general introduction to the same material, see Theodore R. Marmor & Jerry Mashaw,
Northern Light: Canada's Lessons for American Health Care, Am. Prospect, Fall
1990, at 18.

88. *See* Robin Toner, *Bad News for Bush as Poll Shows National Gloom,* N.Y.
Times, Jan. 28, 1992, at A1.

89. *See* Arnold S. Relman, *Universal Health Insurance: Its Time Has Come,* 320 New
Eng. J. Med. 117 (1989).

90. *See* David U. Himmelstein et al., *A National Health Program for the United
States,* 320 New Eng. J. Med. 102 (1989).

91. *See* Special Issue, *Caring for the Uninsured and Underinsured,* 265 JAMA 2491
(1991).

92. *See* Theodore R. Marmor, *U.S. Medical-Care System: Why Not the Worst?,* Wall
St. J., June 20, 1991, at A15; Theodore R. Marmor et al., *Political Handcuffs
Hobble Debate,* L.A. Times, Oct. 3, 1991, at B7.

99. *See* Henry J. Aaron, Serious and Unstable Condition: Financing America's Health
Care 130–31 (1991).

94. *See id.* at 124–28; Marmor & Mashaw, *supra* note 87, at 18–29; Ronald Pollack &
Phyllis Torda, *The Pragmatic Road toward National Health Insurance,* Am. Prospect, Summer 1991, at 92, 95; Paul Starr, *The Middle Class and National Health
Reform,* Am. Prospect, Summer 1991, at 7, 11–12. *But see* Joe White, *Why Congress Should Push a National Health Plan,* Wash. Post, Sept. 15, 1991, at C3
(arguing that a Canadian-style plan is more efficient and politically feasible).

CHAPTER 6: RATIONING

1. National Center for Health Statistics. *Health: United States, 1983.* Hyattsville, Md.: DHHS Pub. No. (PHS) 84–1232, pp. 185–186, 1983.
2. Robert M. Gibson, Daniel R. Waldo, and Katherine R. Levit. "National Health Expenditures, 1982." *Health Care Financing Review* (Fall 1983): 1.
3. National Center for Health Statistics. *Health: United States, 1984.* Hyattsville, Md.: DHHS Pub. No. (PHS) 85–1232, Table 72, p. 137, 1984.
4. Mark S. Freeland and Carol E. Schendler. "Health Spending in the 1980's." *Health Care Financing Review* (Spring 1984): 7.
5. *Health: United States, 1983,* pp. 306, 364.
6. "Increased Migration of Physicians to Rural Areas Seen for Next Decade." *Hospitals* 58, no. 4 (1984): 31.
7. Katherine Swartz, testimony before Subcommittee on Health, Committee on Finance, U.S. Senate, on health care for the economically disadvantaged, April 27, 1984.
8. Robert Wood Johnson Foundation, "Updated Report on Access to Health Care for the American People," *Special Report* (no. 1), 1983.
9. W. B. Schwartz, "The Most Painful Prescription," *Newsweek* (Nov. 12, 1984): 24.
10. H. J. Aaron, and W. B. Schwartz. *The Painful Prescription: Rationing Health Care.* Washington, D.C.: Brookings, 1984.
11. *Id.* at 13.
12. See for instance, Harry Eckstein, *The English Health Service* (Cambridge, Mass.: Harvard University Press, 1959); and A. J. Willcocks, *The Making of the National Health Service* (London: Routledge, Kegan and Paul, 1967).
13. H. J. Aaron, and W. B. Schwartz. "Rationing Hospital Care: Lessons from Britain," *New England Journal of Medicine* 310 (1984): 52–56.
14. *Painful Prescription,* p. vii.
15. Robert B. Evans, *Strained Mercy: The Economics of Canadian Health Care* (Toronto: Butterworths, 1984).
16. *Painful Prescription,* p. 8.
17. R. Klein, "Strategies for Comparative Social Policy Research," in A. Williamson and G. Room, eds. *Health and Welfare States of Britain* (London: Heineman Educational Books, 1983; and T. R. Marmor, A. Bridges, and W. L. Hoffman. "Comparative Politics and Health Policies: Notes on Benefits, Costs, Limits," in D. E. Ashford, ed., *Comparing Public Policies: New Concepts and Methods* (Beverly Hills, Calif.: Sage Publications, 1978), pp. 59–80.
18. Committee on Economic Security, *Report to the President* (Washington, D.C.: U.S. Government Printing Office, 1935).
19. H. L. Wilensky, *The Welfare State and Equality* (Berkeley: University of California Press, 1975); P. Flora, J. Alber, and J. Kohl, "Zur Entwicklung des West-Europaischen Wohlfahrtsstaaten." *Politische Vierteljahresschrift* 18 (4), 1977; J. Carrier and I. Kendall, "The Development of Welfare States: The Production of Plausible Accounts." *Journal of Social Policy* 6 (July 1977).

20. H. Eckstein, *Pressure Group Politics* (London: Allen and Unwin, 1960).
21. T. R. Marmor, and D. Thomas. "Doctors, Politics and Pay Disputes." *British Journal of Political Science* 2 (1972):421–442.
22. *Painful Prescription,* pp. 120–121.
23. *Painful Prescription,* p. 123.
24. *Painful Prescription,* p. 9.
25. *Painful Prescription,* p. 7.
26. *Painful Prescription,* p. 134.
27. *Painful Prescription,* p. 7.
28. G. B. Rosenfeld, Testimony before Select Committee on Aging, U.S. House of Representatives, on "An International Perspective on Health Care," May 1, 1984.

CHAPTER 7: AMERICAN MEDICAL CARE REFORM

1. Philip J. Hilts, "U.S. Health Bill Expected to Rise by 11% for '91," *New York Times,* 30 December 1991.
2. In 1989, an estimated 33.4 million Americans (13.6 percent) had no health insurance. Of the uninsured, 25.6 percent were children. Committee on Ways and Means, U.S. House of Representatives, *Overview of Entitlement Programs: 1991 Green Book* (Washington, D.C.: U.S. Government Printing Office, 1991), 307. The number of Americans without health insurance during the course of an entire year is obviously larger than the cited figure because people move in and out of insurance status. For a variety of estimates of the uninsured, see Emily Friedman, "The Uninsured: From Dilemma to Crisis," *JAMA* 265 (1991): 2491.
3. Sixty percent of Americans were insured through employer plans, while another 12.8 percent were covered under Medicare, 6.0 percent under Medicaid, and 7.7 percent through CHAMPUS, individually purchased policies, or other sources. Committee on Ways and Means, *1991 Green Book,* 309.
4. See Emily Friedman, "Insurers under Fire," *Health Management Quarterly* 13 (3) (1991): 23–24; U.S. General Accounting Office, *Health Insurance: Cost Increases Lead to Coverage Limitations and Cost Shifting* (Washington, D.C.: General Accounting Office, 1990).
5. Friedman, "Insurers under Fire," 26.
6. Paul Cotton, "Preexisting Conditions 'Hold Americans Hostage' to Employers and Insurance," *JAMA* 265 (1991): 2451.
7. Cynthia Sullivan and Thomas Rice, "The Health Insurance Picture in 1990," *Health Affairs* 10 (Summer 1991): 113.
8. Robert Kerrey, "Why America Will Adopt Comprehensive Health Care Reform," *American Prospect* (Summer 1991): 85.
9. Regina Herzlinger, "Healthy Competition," *Atlantic Monthly* (August 1991): 71.
10. Robert J. Blendon and Humphrey Taylor, "Views on Health Care: Public Opinion in Three Nations," *Health Affairs* 8 (1) (1989): 149–57.
11. See Paul Starr, *The Logic of Health Care Reform* (Nashville, Tenn.: Whittle Publications, 1992).

12. For a detailed description, see Theodore R. Marmor and Jerry L. Mashaw, "Northern Light: Canada's Lessons for American Health Care," *American Prospect* (Fall 1990): 18–29; General Accounting Office, *Canadian Health Insurance: Lessons for the United States* (Washington, D.C.: GAO, 1991).

13. For a more detailed discussion of such plans, see Theodore R. Marmor and Michael S. Barr, "Making Sense of the National Health Insurance Reform Debate," *Yale Law & Policy Review* 10 (2) (1992).

14. Alain C. Enthoven, "Consumer-Centered vs. Job-Centered Health Insurance," *Harvard Business Review* (January–February 1979): 147.

15. Ibid., 144–45.

16. Robert G. Evans, "'Rationing' Health Care: The Loaded Alternative," *Frontiers of Health Service Management* (Fall 1987): 31.

17. For a thoughtful elaboration of this point, see Rudolph Klein, "Dilemmas and Decisions," *Health Management Quarterly* 14 (2) (1992): 2–5; see also the symposium on rationing published in the *University of Pennsylvania Law Review* 140 (2) (1992).

18. Joseph A. Califano, Jr., "Rationing Health Care: The Unnecessary Solution," *University of Pennsylvania Law Review* 1526.

19. Even here, it is worth being a bit skeptical; consider the story of the Swedish Dr. Svenson. He arrives at his office Monday morning to find a 94-year-old male patient frenetically seeking his counsel. The patient, waving a copy of the American Surgeon General's report on health promotion, asks: "Is it true what I read here? If I give up chocolate, cut down on red meat, increase my consumption of fiber, forgo sex, mixed drinks, and french fries, and walk two miles a day, will I really live 3.4 years longer than I otherwise would?" Dr. Svenson is reported to have replied: "I don't know about the science of this prediction, but it will *seem longer*." Attributed to Professor Odin Anderson, Department of Sociology, University of Wisconsin.

20. Louise Russell, *Is Prevention Better than Cure?* (Washington, D.C.: Brookings, 1986).

21. For a more detailed discussion of the similarities and differences among precompetitive plans, see Marmor and Barr, "Making Sense of the National Health Insurance Reform Debate."

22. Enthoven, "Consumer-Centered vs. Job-Centered Health Insurance," 147.

23. Starr, "The Logic of Health Care Reform."

24. See Humphrey Taylor and Robert Leitman, "Consumers' Satisfaction with Their Health Care," in Robert J. Blendon and Jennifer N. Edwards, eds., *System in Crisis: The Case for Health Care Reform* (Washington, D.C.: Faulkner & Gray's, 1991), 75–102.

25. Quoted in Theodore Marmor and Jerry Mashaw, "Checking the Nation's Pulse: America's Health Insurance Fever," *Washington Post,* November 17, 1991.

26. Henry Aaron, "Why Bother? America Won't Buy It," *Washington Post,* September 15, 1991.

27. See Theodore R. Marmor, "Coping with a Creeping Crisis: Medicare at Twenty,"

in Theodore R. Marmor and Jerry L. Mashaw, eds., *Social Security: Beyond the Rhetoric of Crisis* (Princeton: Princeton University Press, 1988), 179.

28. The 1992 presidential campaign only exacerbated this tendency. For months, President Bush rarely promoted his own reform plan, offering instead demagogic attacks on "government-run health insurance" (which he on various occasions analogized to the KGB). The approach was clearly designed to portray the Democrats as agents of "socialized medicine"; indeed, some Republican strategists admitted as much. Bill McInturff, a political consultant advising the Bush campaign, conceded that "ads you will see will not be fair, appropriate, or accurate. . . . But let the Democrats try to explain." (Tom Hamburger, "Debate on Health care Suffers from Serious Ailment: Politics," *Minneapolis Star and Tribune*, August 30, 1992). As of September 15, 1992, the Clinton campaign had not settled on a specific reform proposal, although Clinton pledged commitment to universal coverage and the control of medical costs. At various times, Clinton praised play-or-pay plans, mandated universal insurance ("play"), and the merits of "managed competition." What is clear is that the Clinton campaign anticipated Republican distortions in refraining from a detailed plan of its own.

CHAPTER 8: REFLECTIONS ON THE ARGUMENT FOR COMPETITION IN MEDICAL CARE

1. U.S. Bureau of the Census, *Statistical Abstract of the United States: 1990*, 110th ed. (Washington, D.C.: U.S. Government Printing Office), 92 (Table 134). Frequently ignored in expressed concern about the overall cost of health care was (and is) the more important question of the marginal benefit derived from each additional dollar of health spending. Although the assumption is often made that the goods and services purchased in the name of health care remain the same over time, this assumption overlooks the profound changes in medical technology and practice that have occurred in the past 20 years.

2. It may be hard to remember, but at one time economics helped to provide justification for government intervention and regulation: "The principal motive for the increased application of economics to public policy after World War II was the expanding of government as a purveyor of large public programs entailing major expenditures." Evan M. Melhado, "Competition versus Regulation in American Health Policy," in *Money, Power, and Health Care*, Evan M. Melhado, Walter Feinberg, and Harold M. Swartz, eds. (Ann Arbor: Health Administration Press, 1988), p. 35.

3. Melhado, "Competition versus Regulation," pp. 41–45.

4. Melhado, "Competition versus Regulation," p. 87*n*65.

5. According to the *New York Times*, national health expenditures as measured by the Commerce Department rose 11 percent from November 1990 to November 1991 to a total of $738 billion. Outlays of approximately $817 billion were forecast for 1992, 14 percent of predicted GNP. New York Times, December 30, 1991, p. A10.

Actual outlays for 1991 were $838.5 billion, representing 13.2 percent of GNP, as compared with 1992 expenditures of $939.9 billion, or 14 percent of GNP. New York Times, January 5, 1993, A-1, A-10.

6. See, for example, "Dialogue: The Great Health Care Debate: Will Managed Competition Work?" *New York Times,* January 25, 1992, Section 1, p. 23.

7. Alain C. Enthoven and Richard Kronick, "Universal Health Insurance through Incentives Reform," *Journal of the American Medical Association* 265 (May 15, 1991):2532.

8. For a discussion of the hopes and philosophies underlying the antitrust approach see T. R. Marmor, Richard Boyer, and Julie Greenberg, "Medical Care and Pro-competitive Reform," *Vanderbilt Law Review* 34 (1981):1003–28.

9. see A. Enthoven and R. Kronick, "A Consumer Choice Health Plan for the 1990s: Universal Health Insurance in a System Designed to Promote Quality and Economy: I and II," *New England Journal of Medicine* 320 (1989):29–37, 94–101.

10. Data for 1987–1989 from the Group Health Association of America's Annual HMO Industry Survey as cited in Marsha R. Gold, "HMOs and Managed Care," *Health Affairs* (Winter 1991):196.

11. Eli Ginzberg, "U.S. Health Policy—Expectations and Realities," *Journal of the American Medical Association* (December 23/30, 1988):3648.

12. Gold, "HMOs and Managed Care," p. 193.

13. Alain C. Enthoven, "Consumer-Centered vs. Job-Centered Health Insurance," *Harvard Business Review* (January/February 1979):147.

14. See Norman Daniels, *Just Health Care* (Cambridge: Cambridge University Press, 1985).

15. D. Callahan, "Allocating Health Resources," *Hastings Center Report* 18 (1988):14–20; quoted in Charles E. Oswalt, "Expensive Health Care: A Solvable Problem?" in *Archives of Internal Medicine* 150 (1990):1165.

16. T. B. Fitzpatrick, "Changes and Choices in the Health Care System," (Cambridge, Mass.: Cambridge Reports Inc., 1987); as cited in Blendon and Edwards, *System in Crisis,* pp. 35–88.

17. L. Harvey, *AMA Surveys of Physician and Public Opinion: 1986* (Chicago: American Medical Association, 1986).

18. Regina Herzlinger, "Healthy Competition," *Atlantic,* August 1991, p. 71.

19. Others have articulated the skepticism of this chapter with striking clarity. See, for instance, the claims of James Morone and Lawrence D. Brown in companion chapters to ours published earlier in a special volume on *Competitive Approaches to Health Care Reform,* edited by Richard J. Arnoud, Robert F. Rich, and William D. White (Washington, D.C.: Urban Institute Press, 1993).

Morone, in a well-crafted essay on "The Ironic Flaw in Health Care Competition: The Politics of Markets," notes that the success of competitive proposals ironically depends on the capacity of skillful government regulators to set the right rules and enforce them. "Although health care regulation is rooted in a skeptical view of government," he points out, "to succeed, competition requires extraordinarily careful and sophisticated government" (p. 208). The great irony, he rightly emphasizes, is that "health care competition is only as good as the government that competition advocates have so long and loudly deprecated" (p. 212).

Brown's essay, "Competition and the New Accountability," extends irony into paradox. He highlights the greatest paradox of the procompetition movement in American health care reform: namely, "How did we move from policies declaring allegiance to competition to what is becoming the most clinically regulated system in the world?" (p. 223).

These two essays, it should be obvious, provide independent support for the argument of this chapter.

CHAPTER 9: THE CASE FOR STRAIGHTFORWARD REFORM

1. R. J. Blendon and H. Taylor, "Views on Health Care: Public Opinion in Three Nations," *Health Affairs* 8 (1989): 149–157.
2. For a range of estimates, see E. Friedman, "The Uninsured: From Dilemma to Crisis", *J. of the American Medical Assoc.* 265 (1991): 2491–95.
3. R. J. Blendon, "Three Systems: A Comparative Survey," *Health Management Quarterly* 11 (1989): 2–10.
4. H. Taylor and U. Reinhardt, "Does the System Fit?" *Health Management Quarterly* 13 (1991): 2.
5. R. J. Blendon, R. Leitman, I. Morrison, and K. Donelan, "Satisfaction with Health Systems in Ten Nations," *Health Affairs* 9 (1990): 185–192.
6. For a historical account of the debate on national medical care, see P. Starr, *The Social Transformation of American Medicine* (New York: Basic Books, 1982).
7. In 1991, total health expenditures in the United States were estimated at $740 billion. See P. Hilts, "U.S. Health Bill Expected to Rise by 11% for '91," *New York Times,* December 30, 1991.
8. The U.S. Department of Commerce put the 1992 total at $838.5 billion. See R. Pear, "Health-Care Costs Up Sharply Again, Posing New Threat," *New York Times,* January 5, 1992.
9. D. Himmelstein and S. Woolhandler, "Cost without Benefit: Administrative Waste in U.S. Health Care," *New England J. of Medicine* 314 (1986): 441.
10. For an estimate of savings and administrative costs were the United States to shift to universal coverage, see the report by the General Accounting Office, *Canadian Health Insurance: Lessons for the United States* (Washington, D.C.: GAO, 1991).
11. S. Woolhandler and D. Himmelstein, "The Deteriorating Administrative Efficiency of the U.S. Health Care System," *New England* J. of Medicine 324 (1991): 1253.
12. See, e.g., B. Gray, *The Profit Motive and Patient Care* (Cambridge, Mass.: Harvard University Press, 1991).
13. Quoted in T. Marmor and J. Mashaw, "Checking the Nation's Pulse: America's Health Insurance Fever," *Washington Post,* November 17, 1991.
14. T. Marmor, "Misleading Notions: Social, Political, and Economic Myths Prevent Us from Learning from Other Countries' Experiences in Financing Health Care," *Health Management Quarterly* 13 (1991): 18–24.

15. K. R. Levit, H. C. Lazenby, S. W. Letsch, and C. A. Cowan, "National Health Care Spending," *Health Affairs* 10 (1989): 117–130. Quoted in S. T. Sonnefeld, D. R. Waldo, J. A. Lemieux, and D. R. McKusick, "Projections of National Health Expenditures through the Year 2000," *Health Care Financing Review* 13 (1991): 1.

16. M. Peterson, "Political Influence in the 1990's: From Iron Triangles to Policy Networks," *J. of Health Politics, Policy and Law* 18 (1993): 395–438.

17. For a thoughtful elaboration of this point, see R. Klein, "Dilemmas and Decisions," *Health Management Quarterly* 14 (1992): 2–5.

18. For a more detailed discussion of two dominant models of health insurance in other advanced industrialized countries, see T. Marmor and M. Barr, "Making Sense of the National Health Insurance Reform Debate," *Yale Law and Policy Review* 10, no. 2 (1992).

19. E. Ryten, "Medical Schools in Canada," *J. of the American Medical Assoc.* 258 (1987): 1093.

20. Internal Accounting Office, *Canadian Health Insurance,* pp. 16, 52.

21. H. Aaron, "Why Bother? America Won't Buy It," *Washington Post,* September 15, 1991.

22. J. I. Morrison, "Visions, Values and Impediments," *Health Management Quarterly* 13 (1991): 15, 17–18.

23. *The President's Comprehensive Health Reform Program* (1992).

24. See the Mitchell-Kennedy-Riegle-Rockefeller bill, known as "Americare," S.1227, 102nd Congress (1991).

25. See T. Marmor, "Coping with a Creeping Crisis: Medicare at Twenty," in T. Marmor and J. Mashaw, eds., *Social Security: Beyond the Rhetoric of Crisis* (Princeton: Princeton University Press, 1988), p. 179.

26. H. Aaron, *Serious and Unstable Condition: Financing America's Health Care* (Washington, D.C.: Brookings, 1991); and W. Schwartz, "The Inevitable Failure of Current Cost-Containment Strategies: Why They Can Provide Only Temporary Relief," *J. of the American Medical Assoc.* 257 (1987): 220–224.

27. R. G. Evans et al., "Controlling Health Expenditures: The Canadian Reality," *New England J. of Medicine* 320 (1989): 571–577.

28. These basic principles allow for regional variation, but the Canadian Health Act ensures that major departures from these principles result in a dollar-for-dollar reduction in federal aid. Canada Health Act, ch. 6, 15 (1), 1984 S.C.

CHAPTER 12: PATTERNS OF FACT AND FICTION IN USE OF THE CANADIAN EXPERIENCE

1. For a discussion of the contemporary debate over universal health insurance—and the odd place of "managed competition" within it—see the special issue of *Yale Law & Policy Review,* Vol. 10, No. 2 (1992) and, in particular, my essay with Michael S. Barr, "Making Sense of the National Health Insurance Reform Debate." For a thoughtful discussion of the ideas of managed competition, see the last chapter of Paul Starr, *The Logic of Health Care Reform* (Nashville, Tenn.:

Whittle Publications, 1992) and the essays of Starr and Marmor in *American Prospect,* no. 12 (Winter 1993). The literature on managed competition is extensive, but almost entirely hortatory; the journalism is puzzled and confused.

2. Spyros Andreopoulos, ed., *National Health Insurance: Can We Learn from Canada?* (New York: John Wiley, 1975). The sequel to this work, *Medicare at Maturity,* edited by R. G. Grant and W. Stoddart (Calgary: University of Calgary Press, 1984), is far less well known, published as it was during the Reagan years.

3. For an elaboration of this argument, see T. R. Marmor, J. L. Mashaw, and P. L. Harvey, *America's Misunderstood Welfare State* (New York: Basic Books, 1992), especially chapter 6. For more specific North American medical care comparisons, see chapter 10, "On Being Old and Sick: The Burden of Health Care for the Elderly in Canada in the United States," by M. Barer and C. Hertzman in the forthcoming Economic Security and *Intergenerational Justice: A Look at North America,* ed. Marmor, Smeeding, Greene, and Chassman (Washington: Urban Institute, 1994), a project supported by the Donner Foundation.

4. In fairness, the AMA retreated from its propaganda attacks in 1989 after receiving serious criticism from both Canadian physicians and American groups. By 1992 the AMA was taking a far more considered position on universal health insurance, leaving the HIAA as the leading pressure group critical of Canadian Medicare.

5. See, for example, Seymour Martin Lipset, *Continental Divide: The Values and Institutions in the United States and Canada* (New York: Routledge, 1990).

6. See especially the relevant work on North American values by U. Reinhardt and H. Taylor in *Health Management Quarterly* (Fall 1991). For an example of an exchange of letters about Canadian-U.S. cultural differences between Alain Enthoven and Mashaw and Marmor, see *American Prospect,* No. 5 (Spring 1991): 20–24.

7. David U. Himmelstein and Steffie Woolhandler, "A National Health Program for the United States: A Physician's Proposal," *New England Journal of Medicine,* Vol. 320 (January 1989): 102–108.

8. Edward Neuschler, "Canadian Health Care: The Implication of Public Health Insurance," *Health Insurance Association of America Research Bulletin* (Washington, D.C.: HIAA, 1990).

9. *New York Times,* May 30, 1991, p. 25.

10. Reported in T. R. Marmor and Jerry Mashaw, "Canada's Health Insurance and Ours: The Real Lessons, the Big Choices," *American Prospect,* No. 3 (Fall 1990): 18–29, and not denied in an exchange of letters in the subsequent issue of the journal.

11. Lipset, *Continental Divide.*

12. T. R. Marmor, "The Future of American Medical Care," testimony before the Joint Economic Committee of the Congress of the United States, October 2, 1991.

CHAPTER 13: JAPAN—A SOBERING LESSON

1. Notable exceptions are M. Powell and M. Anesaki, with their *Health Care in Japan* (New York: Routledge, 1990).

2. N. Ikegami, "The Japanese Health Care Financing and Delivery System: Its Experiences and Lessons for Other Nations," paper delivered at the International Symposium on Health Care Systems, Taiwan,December 18–19, 1989: 21.

3. Ibid., 26.

4. Powell and Anesaki, *Health Care in Japan*, 128.

5. Ikegami, "Japanese Health Care Financing," 9.

6. Ibid., 17.

7. Ibid., 54.

8. Powell and Anesaki, *Health Care in Japan*, 202.

9. Ikegami, "Japanese Health Care Financing," 10.

10. Powell and Anesaki, *Health Care in Japan*, 128.

11. U.S. Bureau of the Census, *Statistical Abstract of the United States: 1991* (Washington, D.C.: Government Printing Office, 1991): 93.

12. Ikegami, "Japanese Health Care Financing," 10.

13. Drawn from a poll commissioned by the Harvard Community Health Center, December 1991.

14. D. Gross, "Mysteries of the Orient: The Japanese and Health Care Financing," *Health Affairs* 9 (Winter 1990): 219–220.

15. G. Schieber, J. P. Poullier, L. M. Greenwald, "Health Care Systems in Twenty-Four Countries," *Health Affairs* 10 (Fall 1991): 24.

16. Powell and Anesaki, *Health Care in Japan*, 119.

17. Ikegami, "Japanese Health Care Financing," 22.

CHAPTER 15: IMPLEMENTATION

1. See Paul Starr, *The Logic of Health Care Reform* (Nashville, Tenn.: Whittle Publications, 1992), chapter 1.

2. See especially Theodore R. Marmor and David Boyum, "American Medical Care Reform: Are We Doomed to Fail?", *Daedalus,* Vol. 121, No. 4 (Fall 1992); and our "Political Considerations of Competition in Health Care" in *Competitive Approaches to Health Care Reform,* ed. R. Arnould, R. Rich, and W. White (Washington: Urban Institute, 1993).

3. Al From, "What's a New Democrat?" *Washington Post,* June 6, 1993, p. C1.

4. See, for example, the discussion of experience with private health insurance and its adaptability to universal programs in Judy Feder and John Holohan, "Administrative Choices," in Feder, Holohan, and Marmor, *National Health Insurance: Conflicting Goals and Policy Choices* (Washington, D.C.: Urban Institute, 1980), chapter 1, especially pp. 62–69.

5. The Dutch experience bears directly on implementation issues raised by proposals to adjust capitation rates in managed care plans to expected risks. Health experts recognize the enormous variations in use rates both between demographic categories (the old and the young, the rich and the poor) and within them. These variations create opportunities for risk selection by prepaid practice groups (and others) that enroll clients and receive capitation payments on their behalf.

In theory, the right answer is to adjust per capita payments to take into account large differences between broad categories such as men and women or the young and the old. Risk-adjusted capitation rates nonetheless generate enormous problems of implementation. Variations remain substantial within any easily administered adjustments, and more complex adjustments are hard to make, administratively cumbersome, and still open to gaming. The Dutch have discovered this as they wrestle with their form of managed competition, and Medicare administrators know the problems of cream-skimming from their experiences with health maintenance organizations. The debate over managed competition has not addressed this issue of implementation seriously. It should.

6. I mention only in passing the presumption that reducing the tax deductibility of coverage beyond the basic benefit package would substantially affect the decisions of American firms and citizens. This presumption is an excellent example of conflating incentives and behavior, a topic explored in Chapter 7 of Theodore R. Marmor, Jerry L. Mashaw, and Philip L. Harvey, *America's Misunderstood Welfare State* (New York: Basic Books, 1992). The economists who make this claim, and the policy commentators like From who repeat it, have little empirical basis for their presumption. They are correct in noting that treating fringe benefits as taxable provides an incentive to shift income to that category from taxable wages and salaries. But does this make a big difference to either firms or employees? One would have thought that thorough study of the differences between Canada and the United States was called for, since Canada in the period of private insurance expansion after World War II treated health insurance benefits as taxable income and the United States did not. It is noteworthy, but not conclusive, that the North American rate of increase in medical expenditures was practically uniform during the period from 1945 to 1970. It diverged only when Canadian national health insurance completed in 1971 the change in how doctors and hospitals were budgeted and paid—suggestive evidence that changes in the tax treatment of health insurance are, so to speak, marginal. Insurance coverage and payment rules seem the main matters. As a colleague vividly predicted, "Changes in the tax treatment of 'excess' insurance will not produce one less prostate operation. It may well be equitable tax policy to do so, but it is hardly decisive to cost control."

7. There is an exceedingly contentious and confused debate on the truth of this proposition. I will not argue it here, but refer readers to the decade of work by Jean-Pierre Poullier and George Schieber to document this rather obvious point.

8. For evidence of that, see Marilyn Moon, *Medicare Now and the Future* (Washington, D.C.: Urban Institute, 1993), p. 18.

Glossary

ACCOUNTABLE HEALTH PLANS
Programs, usually associated with so-called MANAGED-COMPETITION proposals, that would provide medical coverage to groups of subscribers at variable rates. Such plans would offer a standard benefits package and would issue reports about patient care. The "open" version, for those employed by small companies, would provide coverage through a private administrative body (a HEALTH INSURANCE PURCHASING COOPERATIVE, or HIPC) that would pool individuals for purposes of purchasing insurance. The "closed" plan, for large companies, would not involve an HIPC. These plans are associated with President Clinton's 1993 health reform proposal, as well as with other bills.

ACUTE CARE
Medical care of limited duration for an injury or short-term illness. A doctor usually provides the care in an office or hospital.

ADMINISTRATIVE COSTS
Nonmedical expenditures for health care management (for example, billing, claims processing, marketing, and overhead). Included are (a) the direct costs of insurance managers; (b) the indirect costs paid by other providers for such activities; (c) the nonmonetary costs to patients of dealing with insurance eligibility and billing

ADVERSE SELECTION
The process whereby individuals who know they are most at risk of needing to file an insurance claim disproportionately purchase insurance.

255

AID TO FAMILIES WITH DEPENDENT CHILDREN (AFDC)
A joint federal-state program (sometimes called welfare) that provides grants to those low-income individuals and their dependent children who meet eligibility requirements.

ALLIANCE FOR HEALTH REFORM (AHR)
A nonprofit organization that coordinates conferences and distributes information regarding health care reform; founded in 1991 by Senator John D. Rockefeller IV (D., W.Va.).

ALLIANCE FOR MANAGED COMPETITION
A lobbying organization formed by the major health insurance companies

ALL-PAYER SYSTEM
A system of reimbursement under which government and private insurance plans ("all payers") pay the same amount for the same service. For instance, federal-state MEDICAID insurance programs would not be able to reimburse hospitals at a lower rate than a private insurer such as BLUE CROSS. The health provider thus could not shift costs from one payer to another.

AMBULATORY CARE
Services provided to individuals who are not inpatients in a health care institution.

AMERICAN ASSOCIATION OF RETIRED PERSONS (AARP)
A lobbying group for individuals aged 50 or older. Founded in 1958, it currently has 33 million members.

AMERICAN HEALTH SECURITY ACT
The name of the legislation that President Clinton proposed to Congress in 1993 to "reform" the provision and financing of U.S. medical care.

AMERICAN HOSPITAL ASSOCIATION (AHA)
A trade association representing hospitals, health care facilities, and medical administrators. Founded in 1898, today it has 50,000 members.

AMERICAN MEDICAL ASSOCIATION (AMA)
An organization founded in 1847 that currently represents 297,000 of this country's 600,000 doctors.

BAD DEBT AND FREE CARE
Both terms apply to hospital bills that are not paid. Free care refers to the bills of those too poor to be expected to pay. Bad debt refers to bills left unpaid by those who reasonably might be expected to pay.

BENEFITS
See Health benefits.

BLUE CROSS/BLUE SHIELD ASSOCIATION
The nonprofit national organization of 69 independent corporations that constitute the oldest and largest private health insurer in the United States and the largest

THIRD-PARTY administrator of MEDICARE benefits. Its affiliates provide health insurance to more than 67.5 million Americans.

CALIFORNIA PUBLIC EMPLOYEES' RETIREMENT SYSTEM (CalPERS)

Employing one approach to MANAGED COMPETITION, CalPERS organizes pension, health, and other benefits for state and local government workers in California. It negotiates prices with nineteen HEALTH MAINTENANCE ORGANIZATIONS (HMOS) and four PREFERRED PROVIDER ORGANIZATIONS (PPOS) and monitors the quality of care. With 890,000 members, CalPERS is the largest state health system.

CANADIAN PLAN

The national health insurance system—administered by the ten provinces—that covers the hospital care, outpatient care, and some prescription drugs for all Canadians. Usually called a SINGLE-PAYER SYSTEM, Canada's "Medicare" is financed 38 percent by national taxation and 62 percent by provincial taxation. Private doctors in FEE-FOR-SERVICE practices bill the provincial health ministries monthly; community-owned hospitals negotiate annual budgets with the provincial governments. The provincial governments set rates limiting the fees that providers can charge.

CAPITATION

A payment method in which a doctor or hospital is paid a fixed amount per patient per year—regardless of the services used by the patient. The method is typically used by American HMOS, but is also the way most British general practitioners are paid.

CASE MANAGEMENT

One way of handling patients in MANAGED CARE systems; also known as gatekeeping. In PRIMARY-CARE case management, a practitioner determines how much and what kinds of service (including that of specialists) a patient requires. ACUTE-CARE case management usually deals with high-cost, seriously ill patients; a case manager monitors services and can arrange for alternative treatments. The system is sometimes regarded as meddlesome, sometimes as helpful.

CATASTROPHIC COVERAGE

Insurance that pays for very large health care expenses (usually associated with accidents or chronic illnesses and diseases, such as cancer and AIDS). In general, this coverage is expensive and hard to find.

CATHOLIC HEALTH ASSOCIATION OF THE UNITED STATES

An umbrella organization for more than 1,200 nonprofit Catholic health care facilities; founded in 1915.

CHAMPUS

An acronym for the Civilian Health and Medical Program of the Uniformed Services. The organization finances the health care of dependents of active-duty military personnel, plus retired military personnel and their dependents. The Department of Defense provides health care directly to active-duty personnel.

CHARITY CARE
Free health care given by doctors, nurses, and hospitals. (In 1956, the Internal
Revenue Service mandated charity care for nonprofit hospitals, to keep their tax-
exempt status; that ruling was rescinded in 1969 but many hospitals continue to
provide free care.)

COBRA
The Consolidated Omnibus Budget Reconciliation Act of 1985. It requires employers to make it possible for individuals who lose their health insurance for various
reasons to continue to purchase such coverage for two years with their own funds,
through the employer's plan.

COINSURANCE
The percentage of medical costs, not covered by insurance, that an individual
must pay. (Many plans pay only 80 percent of hospital and doctor's costs.)

COMMUNITY RATING
A method for determining the price of health insurance premiums (the yearly
amount that individuals pay for coverage). A community rating premium is based
on the average medical cost for all covered people in a geographic area. The system is historically associated with nonprofit BLUE CROSS/BLUE SHIELD plans, most
of which abandoned community rating when forced to compete with commercial
insurers in the 1950s and thereafter.

CONTINUUM OF CARE
A range of services and care settings that patients may require at different stages
of their illness.

COPAYMENT
The fee that must be paid by patients when they use health care—despite their
insurance. Such "copays" range from nominal fees per visit (say, three dollars at
an HMO) to higher preset limits.

COST SHARING
A provision of a health care plan that requires individuals to cover some part of
their medical expenses. It may help to hold down costs by deterring individuals
from seeking unnecessary care, or it may discourage necessary care. In universal
insurance plans, cost sharing is a form of taxation on being sick and using services. Typical forms include DEDUCTIBLES, CO-PAYMENT, and CO-INSURANCE.

DEATH SPIRAL
The term applied when ADVERSE SELECTION gets out of control and sets off suc-
cessive waves of rate increases. At each stage the healthier subscribers drop their
insurance because it has become too expensive—and only those who know they
will need it (those who are sick) retain coverage.

DEDUCTIBLE
The amount a patient must pay out of pocket before health insurance will finance
subsequent costs. (See COST SHARING)

DEFENSIVE MEDICINE
Performing or ordering tests or procedures that would not have otherwise been performed, in order to be able to defend against a potential MALPRACTICE claim.

DIAGNOSIS-RELATED GROUPS (DRGs)
A classification system adopted by MEDICARE in 1983 to set standard Medicare payments for hospitalization. Payments are predetermined based on the patient's diagnosis, having been adjusted for the average cost of such care in the area. After physicians determine the relevant diagnosis, Medicare reimburses the hospital regardless of the particular costs of the beneficiary's hospitalization.

DIRECT EMPLOYER COVERAGE
Health insurance obtained through an individual's employer (current or former), union, or family member. (Sixty percent of Americans are insured through their own employer or that of a family member.)

EMPLOYEE RETIREMENT INCOME SECURITY ACT (ERISA)
A 1974 federal law that set the standards of disclosure for employee benefit plans, to ensure workers the right to at least part of their pension. The law governs most private pensions and other employee benefits, and overrides all state laws that concern employee benefits, including HEALTH BENEFITS. The result has been the exclusion from state insurance regulations of the self-insured health plans of many large companies.

EMPLOYER MANDATE
A requirement that all employers offer and nominally pay for a portion (in the Clinton plan, 80 percent) of their workers' health coverage. Many small businesses seem to fear that a health insurance mandate would be so costly that it would drive them out of business. Most analysts believe that the costs of employer mandates are largely borne by employees.

ENTITLEMENTS
Government benefits, including health care benefits, that are conferred automatically on all qualified individuals. They are part of mandatory spending programs such as Social Security, MEDICARE, MEDICAID, and food stamps. The first two of these programs have a contributory taxation form of finance that underlies the concept of entitlement; the latter two do not.

ERSD
A funding program under MEDICARE for end-stage renal disease that pays for kidney dialysis and kidney transplants.

EXPERIENCE RATING
A method used to determine the price of health insurance premiums based on the amount a certain group (such as the employees of a business) has previously paid for medical services. Indemnity insurance companies most often use experience rating when determining premium rates. Small businesses, however, can be hurt by experience rating, because one employee's severe medical problems can cause a significant increase in the entire group's premiums.

FEE FOR SERVICE
A system of reimbursement in which a medical provider charges a patient (or third-party payer) a specific price for a specific service.

FIRST PARTY
The patient.

FLAT-OF-THE-CURVE MEDICINE
Medical care that produces relatively little or no benefit for the patient as a result of diminishing marginal returns.

FORMULARIES
Lists of approved drugs which are the only ones that can be prescribed by physicians participating in certain programs. The list generally excludes more expensive options when cheaper, equally effective drugs are available.

GENERIC DRUGS
Drugs that are essentially identical to brand-name drugs, without the brand name and without the higher price of the original product.

GLOBAL BUDGET
An amount, set by an administrative body, that controls the funds available to pay for medical care services in a region, state, or nation. Usually covering government spending and other insurance payers, global budgets are most often associated with universal health insurance, under which all individuals in a country are covered.

GROUP HEALTH ASSOCIATION
A trade association made up of the major HMOs.

GUARANTEED NATIONAL BENEFIT PACKAGE
The standard coverage that would be guaranteed to all Americans as a result of President Clinton's proposal.

HEALTH ALLIANCES
Purchasing organizations that, under the Clinton plan, would each buy medical care services for groups of consumers. The alliances would be of two types: regional health alliances, whose creation would be the responsibility of the states, and corporate health alliances. A corporate alliance could be established by any large employer (under the Clinton plan as of February 1994, defined as one with more than five thousand workers). But such an employer would have the option of joining a regional alliance instead.

HEALTH BENEFITS
Payments made by a health insurance firm to patients or medical providers to cover all or some of the costs of medical care.

HEALTH CARE FINANCING ADMINISTRATION (HCFA)
Part of the Department of Health and Human Services, HCFA administers MEDICARE and MEDICAID; it also records Medicare, Medicaid, and national health statistics. Created in 1977.

HEALTH INDUSTRY MANUFACTURERS' ASSOCIATION (HIMA)

A trade association composed of manufacturers of medical devices, diagnostic products, and health care information systems; founded in 1974.

HEALTH INSURANCE ASSOCIATION OF AMERICA (HIAA)

This organization, founded in 1956, represents 270 health insurance firms that write and sell individual and group policies.

HEALTH INSURANCE PURCHASING COOPERATIVE (HIPC)

An HIPC, like a HEALTH ALLIANCE, pools individuals or employees for the purpose of buying health insurance. A health alliance, under the Clinton plan, is quasi-governmental. In other proposals, an HIPC is a private, nonprofit organization.

HEALTH MAINTENANCE ORGANIZATION (HMO)

A prepaid medical care plan in which the organization receives a certain amount (usually monthly), and patients seek treatment from its affiliated medical staff. The goal is to provide affordable health care through forms of MANAGED CARE—in which a PRIMARY-CARE provider is supposed to act as gatekeeper to specialists and expensive medical tests. Often subscribers pay a small amount at each visit. Patients in HMOs have variable limits on their choice of doctors.

Staff model. Doctors are salaried and work only for the HMO, often at a single site.

Group model. Doctors are organized in an independent partnership, corporation, or association that contracts only with the HMO.

Network model. Combines two or more types of HMOs.

HEALTH PLANS

A phrase that has several meanings: (1) the networks of doctors, hospitals, and insurers that would, in the Clinton proposal, provide coverage through contracts negotiated with regional or corporate HEALTH ALLIANCES; (2) the benefits offered by health insurance providers to individuals and companies; (3) methods of paying for health care.

HOLDBACKS

Sums of money due to doctors in an HMO or other MANAGED-CARE system which are not paid until overall volume for the period can be determined. If volume proves to be higher than planned, enough funds are permanently withheld to meet preset expenditure targets.

IATROGENIC INJURY

An injury caused by the process of health care. Not necessarily due to negligence, it may be the result of mistaken policies, bad luck, insufficient skill, and so forth.

INDEMNITY INSURANCE

A traditional health insurance plan in which the patient submits the medical bill to the insurance company for a specified level of reimbursement which may be equal to or less than the fee charged.

INDEPENDENT PRACTICE ASSOCIATION (IPA)
A form of medical practice in which physicians can treat both HMO and private patients. The HMO patients are charged a negotiated rate, usually on a per capita or fixed fee-for-service basis.

INDIRECT EMPLOYER COVERAGE
Insurance provided by an employer to the employees' family members, who may or may not receive fewer benefits than the employees.

INFANT MORTALITY
All deaths of infants (those who are born alive) within the first year of life.

INTEGRATED SERVICE NETWORK (ISN)
A new type of medical plan—one that offers broad medical care coverage—being developed in Minnesota. Quasi-public cooperatives and the state MEDICAID system will negotiate rates and terms with the networks on behalf of large groups of consumers

JACKSON HOLE GROUP
An informal group of business figures and academics who have met for some years at the Jackson Hole, Wyoming, home of Dr. Paul Ellwood to promote their preferred form of health care policy. (Ellwood previously worked for InterStudy, a Minnesota health policy research company.) The group devised the Jackson Hole plan, which calls for ACCOUNTABLE HEALTH PLANS and HEALTH INSURANCE PURCHASING COOPERATIVES. Group members favor what they call MANAGED COMPETITION that incorporates taxation of health benefits above a minimum package.

"JOB LOCK"
Workers remain in a job for fear of losing health insurance coverage altogether, or because a prospective employer's health plan refuses to cover a medical circumstance such as a dependent's PREEXISTING CONDITION.

LONG-TERM CARE
Health care required by chronically ill, physically disabled, or mentally disabled individuals. Such patients usually require round-the-clock supervision in a hospital, nursing home, or (less frequently) at home.

LOSS EXPERIENCE
The amount health insurance companies pay for the health care their policyholders use.

MAJOR MEDICAL
Refers usually to health insurance policies designed to cover substantial expenses associated with serious illness. Typically, policyholders pay extremely high deductibles before coverage starts and may have to pay COINSURANCE as well.

MALPRACTICE
Harmful or unprofessional treatment or neglect of a patient by a doctor or other medical provider.

MANAGED CARE
A type of health care organization that means different things to different people. Sometimes it aims to control costs by using gatekeepers—PRIMARY-CARE doctors or caseworkers—to coordinate the use of medical services by patients. Managed-care networks usually are organized by insurance companies, employers, or hospitals. An example is the type of network run by HMOs, in which a patient sees one doctor who determines the medical care, both general and specialized, that he or she will receive. The patient's access to medical services is thereby controlled.

MANAGED COMPETITION
Both a slogan and a set of ideas about health care reform. Largely embraced by President Clinton as an early label for his reform proposal, it proved a complicated marketing term and was abandoned as a Clinton policy tag. The concept of managed competition combines market forces with government regulation. Large groups of consumers buy medical care (or insurance for care) from networks of providers. The aim is to create price competition among those networks and thereby both restrain prices and encourage high-quality care and responsiveness. The variation among plans described as managed competition is substantial; thus the label is of uncertain worth.

MEDICAID
The federal-state health insurance program for the categorically poor. Enacted in 1965, Medicaid took effect the following year. While program details differ from state to state, all states together spent $50 billion on Medicaid in 1992, and the federal government spent $68 billion. In that year Medicaid paid for the care of 32.6 million people, spending nearly a third of its budget on LONG-TERM CARE.

MEDICAID WAIVER
The formal process by which a state receives federal permission to deviate from certain MEDICAID program rules. The most notorious example of this process involved the state of Oregon's plan to widen Medicaid eligibility while narrowing (RATIONING) the range of services it would finance.

MEDICAL SAVINGS ACCOUNTS
Analogous to individual retirement accounts, but employers and employees can make tax-deferred contributions and employees can withdraw funds to pay covered medical expenses.

MEDICARE
The federal health insurance program for the elderly and disabled enacted in 1965 and started a year later. Its benefits include hospital care, doctor visits, and other services. Financed by individual premiums, social insurance taxes, and general revenues, Medicare is the largest federal health program today, covering not only the elderly but also the disabled and those with chronic renal failure. Largely omitted from the Clinton reform proposal, Medicare expansion is the basis of other proposals—most prominently that of Congressman Fortney (Pete) Stark (D., Calif.).

Part A. The portion of Medicare that pays for hospital care. The program covers inpatient care beyond (in 1992) a $676 deductible and also provides short-term nursing care. Medicare Part A cost $80.8 billion in 1992 and covered 34.4 million people. It is financed by a 1.15 percent payroll tax.

Part B. The so-called voluntary part of Medicare, known as Supplementary Medical Insurance, which pays a portion of doctors' bills. Medicare Part B is supposed to pay 80 percent of a physician's fee, once the beneficiary has met a $100 deductible. Covering 33.6 million people in 1992, Medicare Part B expenditures were $48.6 billion. The program is financed by patient premiums and general federal revenues.

MEDICARE CATASTROPHIC COVERAGE ACT
Passed by Congress in 1988, this law provided benefits for those with catastrophic medical problems, capped out-of-pocket expenses, and covered prescription drugs. But after many senior citizens objected to the new program's financing and rationale, Congress repealed the law in 1989.

MEDIGAP
Private health insurance plans that augment MEDICARE by paying medical bills not covered by the federal government. Payments could include COINSURANCE, coverage of Medicare DEDUCTIBLES, and bills not covered by Medicare (including prescription drugs).

NATIONAL HEALTH BOARD
A seven-member federal panel proposed by President Clinton's reform bill. Appointed by the President to oversee the creation of regional HEALTH ALLIANCES by the states, the board would also be expected to interpret the guaranteed benefits package, enforce a NATIONAL HEALTH CARE budget, monitor the quality of care, and investigate the pricing of new drugs by pharmaceutical companies if evidence suggests that the prices are unreasonably high.

NATIONAL HEALTH BUDGET
The total amount spent on health care by government and private payers. In 1992 the United States spent $832 billion—one-seventh of the entire U.S. economic output. The Congressional Budget Office estimates that the cost may rise to $1.6 trillion by the year 2000.

NATIONAL HEALTH CARE
A misleading label for a health insurance system that covers all citizens and various other residents. Sometimes it is the designation for so-called SINGLE-PAYER version of national health insurance, particularly those modeled after Canada's system. Under such a plan, the government sets all budgets for hospitals and fees for doctors and other providers.

NATIONAL HEALTH SECURITY CARD
An identification card that would serve as proof of a person's eligibility for the government's guaranteed package of benefits. Under the Clinton plan all citizens and legal aliens would be eligible.

OREGON PLAN
See Rationing.

"ORPHAN DRUGS"
Medicines for ailments that afflict fewer than 200,000 people. In 1983 Congress
passed the Orphan Drug Act, which gave tax credits and exclusive market rights
to medical companies involved in developing such drugs. Many considered the law
a success; but critics charged that the law gave drug companies too much latitude
in setting prices and making profits.

PEPPER COMMISSION
A 15-member commission led by the late Representative Claude Pepper (D., Fla.),
which explored how to address the needs of those Americans who lacked health
insurance and how to finance LONG-TERM CARE for the chronically ill or disabled.
In 1990 the commission recommended a PLAY-OR-PAY plan for employers and a
universal plan to cover long-term care services for all Americans.

PER-PERSON PREMIUM
A flat-rate health insurance premium, as opposed to a premium for a family or one
based on a percentage of income.

PHARMACEUTICAL MANUFACTURERS' ASSOCIATION (PMA)
A trade association founded in 1958 that represents 88 companies within the industry that develop and manufacture prescription drugs.

PHYSICIAN PAYMENT REVIEW COMMISSION (PPRC)
Recommends reimbursement rates for doctors in the MEDICARE program. Founded
by Congress in 1986, the 13-member commission is charged with analyzing Medicare payment issues and submitting its findings to Congress. Congress then decides on the policies to be used, and HCFA sets the actual rate.

PLAY OR PAY
A health insurance reform plan in which employers either provide their workers
with a basic HEALTH BENEFITS package ("play") or pay into a government insurance pool. The system was popular in 1991 among congressional Democrats.

POINT-OF-SERVICE PLAN (POS)
A feature of a health insurance plan whereby patients are financially rewarded for
using a limited group of providers, but are permitted to seek out-of-network care
at higher cost.

PREEXISTING CONDITION
A physical or mental condition diagnosed before an individual receives health insurance coverage. Some insurers refuse to cover a person with such a condition;
others increase their rates or refuse to cover the patient for a specific time. Preexisting conditions are the object of intense reform attention in 1994 as an example
of how conventional insurance practices have hurt precisely those who need insurance most.

PREFERRED PROVIDER ORGANIZATION (PPO)
Under this system providers, usually organized by networks or panels, offer medical care for a set fee. Various benefits, such as lower COINSURANCE and better coverage, create incentives for patients to see "preferred" doctors; restrictions on caregivers are, by contrast, the disincentives.

PREMIUM TAX
A state tax on the payments made to an insurance company by policyholders who live in that state.

PRICE CONTROLS
Government-set price ceilings on goods or services. In medical care, the term usually refers to a physician fee schedule.

PRIMARY CARE
The care people routinely receive when they go to the doctor. Primary care can be delivered by a doctor, nurse practitioner, or physician's assistant. Doctors practicing family medicine, pediatrics, or internal medicine are generally considered primary-care providers.

PRIOR APPROVAL
A form of utilization review whereby an insurance company requires a hospital or doctor to get permission from the insurance company before providing care.

PROFILE MONITORING
A process in which the practice patterns of individual physicians are compared to various norms.

PROTOCOL
A guide for the treatment of a specific disease or condition.

QUALIFIED MEDICARE BENEFICIARY
A person aged 65 or older whose income falls below the federal poverty line and for whom the MEDICAID program must pay all MEDICARE costs, including Part B premiums, DEDUCTIBLES, and COPAYMENTS.

RATE SETTING
Refers generally to a government's setting of prices—whether for electricity, water, or health care. Maryland has had such a system for hospitals since the 1970s.

RATIONING
Any process that in medical care limits the services a person can receive. Allocation based on income is widespread in the United States, as are other limits. Rationing is unavoidable in medical care, although the bases of rationing are varied and differently valued.

REINSURANCE
See Stop-loss coverage.

RELATIVE VALUE SCALE (RVS)
A method of establishing differential fees for physicians' services. The RVS was a 1992 effort by MEDICARE to shift funding away from SPECIALISTS, who were receiving relatively high Medicare payments, toward PRIMARY-CARE practitioners. It bases the value of each medical procedure on its complexity. The conversion factor chosen translates the number into a specific dollar amount.

RISK-CONTROL INSURANCE
See Stop-loss coverage.

RISK POOL
A group of people brought together for purposes of pricing insurance. Sometimes the term refers to those who seek insurance but cannot, because of their medical history, get it (a "high" risk pool). In the Clinton plan the risk pool consists of everyone within a HEALTH ALLIANCE or a HEALTH PLAN.

SECOND PARTY
The caregiver or provider. *See also* THIRD-PARTY PAYER.

SELF-INSURANCE
A form of health insurance in which an employer (or others)—but not an insurance company—assumes the risk of health expenses. Third parties may administer such plans.

SINGLE-PAYER OPTION
A provision of the Clinton play that permits a state to choose to make direct payments to medical providers, with no intermediaries

SINGLE-PAYER SYSTEM
A UNIVERSAL COVERAGE plan under which the government collects funds for health insurance and has a uniform plan for everyone in a given state or nation. Canada uses this method of universal health insurance in its ten provinces. The arrangements effectively eliminate private health insurance for basic coverage. Proponents believe it is the best way to reduce substantially the rise in national health costs.

SMALL-GROUP MARKET
Generally, small businesses that employ fewer than 100 employees. The per-employee costs for health insurance are much higher than those of larger firms.

SPECIALIST
Any physician who has pursued specialty training beyond the first year of residency. Often the term implies that the doctor does not provide PRIMARY CARE.

SPEND DOWN
A requirement of many state MEDICAID programs that individuals use up their assets when these are above the level required for eligibility to collect benefits.

STOP-LOSS COVERAGE
Insurance by one insurer of all or part of a risk previously assumed by another insurer (or HEALTH PLAN). It is a form of backup insurance that reimburses a health plan (stops its losses) when the payments it makes exceed the expected outlays. Stop-loss coverage is also known as reinsurance or risk-control insurance.

TASK FORCE ON NATIONAL HEALTH CARE REFORM
The presidential advisory group, formed in January 1993 and chaired by Hillary Rodham Clinton, that worked for four months on a proposed overhaul of the American health care system. The task force comprised more than 500 people, largely technical specialists, drawn from within the government and private organizations.

THIRD PARTY ADMINISTRATOR
A person or corporate entity that handles the administrative details of health insurance for a SELF-INSURED group. The group assumes the financial risks; the third party does not.

THIRD-PARTY PAYER
A person or organization that pays all or part of a set of medical expenses—but not the patient (the first party) or the caregiver (the second party). Examples are MEDICAID, MEDICARE, BLUE CROSS/BLUE SHIELD, and most commercial health insurance companies. An HMO need not involve a third-party payer.

UNCOMPENSATED CARE
Services given by hospitals or other providers that are not paid for by patients, their insurance companies, or the government. The cost of such care is often shifted to paying patients or their insurers.

UNDERINSURED
Those persons—estimated at 15 million to 30 million in the United States—with inadequate health insurance. High DEDUCTIBLES, limited coverage, unavailable providers, and waiting periods are all sources of inadequate coverage.

UNINSURED
Those people without health insurance, estimated in a 1991 Census Bureau study at 36.6 million Americans.

UNIVERSAL COVERAGE
Refers to a situation where all (citizens-residents) have health insurance.

UTILIZATION REVIEW
A process by which an insurance company reviews decisions of doctors and hospitals on what care to provide for patients.

VOLUME PERFORMANCE STANDARDS
The number of physician services that the managers of a HEALTH PLAN expect to be provided in a given period.

WAGE-BASED PREMIUM

Similar to a tax, this method of raising funds for health care requires all employers to pay a percentage of their payroll for their employees' health insurance. A small portion of the premium may be paid by the employee.

WORKERS' COMPENSATION INSURANCE

Insurance that reimburses employers for the costs of compensating employees who are injured in the course of their employment.

Index

Aaron, Henry, 110–17, 135, 152, 167

Abel-Smith, Brian, 26

Access to health care: connected to cost and quality, 14–15, 26, 64, 74, 86, 89, 110, 194; uneven, 22, 24, 46, 73, 74, 109, 187; denied to control costs, 26, 66, 100; and government subsidies, 57, 72; in for-profits, 66–72, 234; in nonprofits, 66–72, 73, 78–79; exclusionary policies, 69–70, 73, 219–20; policy issues, 72–73, 78–79; agreement on universal access, 86, 144, 210; controlled by price, 130, 144; in Japan, 199, 200. *See also* Cream-skimming; Patient selection; Rationing of medical care; Universal coverage

Accountability, 17–18, 126, 151, 158, 189–90, 191, 192–94

Acquired immune deficiency syndrome (AIDS), 89, 96

Acute care, 53, 54, 58, 229

Administrative costs: reform to reduce, 16–17, 221–23; current level, 17; of waste-cutting, 91, 95; of private insurance, 124, 150, 182, 191–92; fear of, 149–50; of managed care, 156, 173–74, 219–20, 222–23; cross-national studies, 168; in Canada, 168, 186, 191–92; of complex reform plans, 213; of price controls, 213; of adjusting for patient risk, 219, 220, 252–53; of single-payer plans, 220, 222

Advertising, 141, 247

Age, as a care criterion, 97. *See also* Elderly

Agency for Health Care Policy and Research (AHCPR), 94, 95, 103, 104, 238–39

Aid to Families with Dependent Children (AFDC), 37–38. *See also* Welfare state

Alliances. *See* Health alliances

Allocation of care. *See* Rationing of medical care

271

Waste cutting (continued)
  effectiveness, 103, 130–31, 236, 242–
  43; policy problems, 103–6. *See also*
  Necessary care; Rules, allocational
Welfare state: international comparisons, 31–32, 38–42, 46–47, 228; international criticism, 32–34, 38, 39,
  180; nature of the "crisis," 33–34,
  46; causes economic problems, 34–
  36; economic problems cause a crisis, 34, 36–37, 42, 43–44; and governmental legitimacy, 34, 37–38; levels of social spending, 35–38, 39–42,

43–44, 228–29; economic assump-
  tions, 36–37, 229; U.S. policies, 40–
  41, 42–44; income elasticity, 40–41,
  229; intergenerational strains, 211–
  12. *See also* Aid to Families with
  Dependent Children
Wellstone, Paul, 11, 160, 182
White, Joseph, 157
Wing, Ken, 27
Wofford, Harris, 4
Woolhandler, Steffie, 166–67

Young, Quentin, 159–60, 164